The Biohackers Guide to Spiritual Bodybuilding

Nahum Justin Vizakis

This book is dedicated to Bostin Lloyd, Dallas McCarver, Rich Piana, and Kristi Enos, May they Rest in Peace. May we all have the inner strength and faith to love ourselves enough to approach Bodybuilding with presence, patience and acceptance, and to pass on these lessons learned so the next generation can show up healthy and whole.

Contents

Foreword: Iron and Insight

I first stepped on stage in 2009, during a deployment to Iraq. It was my debut as a natural competitor, and I had been bodybuilding for less than a year. But the roots of my path in physical culture go much deeper. I had been an athlete for as long as I could remember.

At just 13 years old, I joined my high school powerlifting team. One afternoon in the weight room, I was messing around with a few friends, squatting alongside the varsity football players. The coach noticed my form and approached me. Without hesitation, he told me to load two plates on the bar. At the time, I didn't even know how much that was. But it got everyone's attention. I dropped into a perfect squat—twice—and stood up with ease. That was the moment I realized: I wasn't your average bear when it came to strength and movement. Something deeper lived in me—a potential, a drive, a raw connection to the body that would later become both a gift and a teacher.

When I made the decision to compete, the world looked very different than it does now. There was no Instagram, no TikTok, no endless sea of influencers offering advice. The only place I could find community was the **bodybuilding.com forums**, where a handful of seasoned competitors generously shared their hard-earned wisdom. I still remember buying my first book on nutrition and performance enhancement—**Dan Duchaine's *Underground Body Opus***. It was militant, intense, radical. And for years, it was my bible for cutting, recomposition, and learning the art of manipulating the body with intention.

2009 I competed at Camp Taji Iraq (First place, Overall), 2010 Austin Texas (Texas showdown, Fist place, Overall) 2011 Copper Classic Phoenix AZ (First place, Overall), 2012 San Jose Championship (First Place), LA championships (5th Place) and The USA's Las Vegas (11th Place), 2013 NPC Nationals (33rd Place) and 2022 Jay Cutler Classic (Masters first place), I competed in eight shows. Over the years, the landscape of bodybuilding and fitness has changed dramatically—new science, new substances, new cultural values. And yet, the core remains: this sport still stands as a crucible, forging identity and will, body and mind.

This book is not just a guide to training or nutrition. It's a **contemplation on the soul of bodybuilding**—a synthesis of my years spent on stage, behind the scenes, and within myself. Living in Las Vegas for much of that time gave me an insider's perspective into the fitness industry's highs and lows. I've seen the dysfunction, the addictions, the ego traps. But I've also seen the transformation, the healing, and the sacred potential that emerges when muscle becomes meditation.

My intention in writing this is to illuminate the full spectrum of the path—from the shadow to the sacred. This is for anyone who's ever looked in the mirror and seen more than a body staring back—for those who understand that beneath the steel and sweat lies something far more powerful: **the awakening of the human spirit through discipline, devotion, and self-realization.**

Chapter 1: The Sacred Temple – Reframing the Body

Historical context: bodybuilding as art, discipline, and self-transformation

Bodybuilding, at its surface, may seem to be a purely physical pursuit—an arena of muscle, symmetry, and aesthetics. But beneath the sweat and repetition lies a profound **philosophical architecture**: a way of life built upon discipline, transformation, self-conquest, and even metaphysics. To understand bodybuilding deeply is to recognize it not only as sport or spectacle, but as a **spiritual forge**—a modern form of **ritualized self-mastery**.

Let's walk through its philosophical framework, layer by layer.

🏛 The Temple of the Self (Ontology)

At its core, bodybuilding rests on a radical premise:

The body is both material and malleable.

The sport begins with the assumption that the human body is not fixed—it can be **sculpted, elevated, disciplined into ideal form**. This is a profoundly ontological stance: the body is not merely given; it is **becoming**.

In this way, the gym is the modern **temple**, and the body becomes a **living artifact—** a temple of the self, built not by divine decree but by human will

Discipline as Devotion (Ethics)

Bodybuilding operates through a strict ethic: **discipline**, **consistency**, and **sacrifice**. The bodybuilder willingly embraces discomfort, delay, and repetition—choosing short-term struggle for long-term mastery.

"What you do in private shows up in public."

This reflects a **Stoic ethic**: mastery over appetite, pain, and distraction.

Every rep is a meditation. Every fasted morning a ritual. The gym becomes a **dojo of the will**, where morality is measured in sets and sacrifice.

The Will to Transform (Existentialism)

Like existentialist philosophy, bodybuilding is about **taking responsibility for becoming**. You do not blame genetics, environment, or excuses. You confront yourself.

"The iron never lies." – Henry Rollins

This is the **existential choice**: to create meaning where none is given. The bodybuilder says: *I will carve myself from chaos*. Every pound lifted is a vote for agency over fate.

Aesthetics as Sacred Geometry (Beauty and Symmetry)

Bodybuilding's judging system is based on **symmetry**, **proportion**, **muscle balance**, and **presentation**—which links directly to classical concepts of **ideal beauty** from Greek philosophy.

Think of it this way:

- The **golden ratio**

- The **statues of Apollo**

- Da Vinci's **Vitruvian Man**

These were not just art—they were blueprints of divine proportion. The bodybuilder becomes an **artist**, using flesh instead of marble, dumbbells instead of chisels. The body is not just a vehicle—**it is the masterpiece**.

🜂 Suffering as Alchemy (Transformation Through Pain)

In bodybuilding, **pain is not an enemy—it's a guidepost**. Muscle is broken to be rebuilt. Hunger is endured to reach clarity. Fatigue is a necessary gatekeeper of growth.

This echoes **alchemical and mystical traditions**: the raw material (prima materia) must be burned, broken, and purified to yield gold.

"The furnace of discipline melts the ego into excellence."

Thus, pain becomes not punishment but **initiation**—a passage to higher identity.

🧘 Dualism and Integration (Mind–Body Unity)

Philosophically, bodybuilding collapses the **mind–body divide**. The idea that "you are either a thinker or a jock" is obliterated. In bodybuilding:

- The **mind commands**, and the **body obeys**—and then teaches back.

- **Mental visualization** drives muscular growth (the "mind–muscle connection").

- **Self-image** is both internal and external: how you see yourself **affects how you build yourself**.

Thus, bodybuilding is not narcissism. It is a **dialogue** between spirit and structure—a constant integration.

✺ Legacy and Meaning (Metaphysics)

At the highest level, bodybuilding becomes a meditation on **mortality and transcendence**.

- Muscles decay.

- Titles fade.

- But the transformation lives on in the psyche.

Like the sand mandalas of Tibetan monks—built, admired, and then destroyed—**the point was never permanence**. The point was the sacred act of creation itself.

To bodybuild is to say: *I will shape myself while I can. I will not leave unchanged.*

🏋 Final Philosophy: The Iron Path

Bodybuilding is not just reps and rice, muscle and macros. It is a philosophical architecture built on:

- The assertion of will over entropy

- The belief that beauty can be built

- The commitment to discipline as self-love

- The sacred use of suffering to spark transformation

It is, at its most profound, **the art of becoming through the body**—a modern mythic journey in protein-stained gym clothes.

- The body as a **vessel for Spirit**, not just an object of desire

Contrast: Two Paradigms of Relationship to the Body

The Body as a Vessel for Spirit

- **Viewpoint:** The body is sacred. It is a temporary home for consciousness, a vehicle for awakening, service, and expression of the divine in form.

- **Rooted in:** Spiritual traditions, mysticism, somatic psychology, martial arts, indigenous and esoteric teachings

- **Focus:** Connection, presence, embodiment, energy flow, alignment with purpose and nature

- **Relationship to Pain:** Seen as a teacher and signal, not a barrier to be overridden

- **Training Motivation:** Cultivation of awareness, discipline, and inner harmony. Lifting becomes a **ritual**, a moving meditation.

"I train not to conquer my body, but to *meet it*—to listen, honor, and refine the instrument through which my soul speaks."

The Body as an Object of Desire

- **Viewpoint:** The body is a project to be perfected, displayed, and used for social capital, pleasure, dominance, or personal validation.

- **Rooted in:** Consumer culture, media, vanity metrics, and the ego's need for identity and control

- **Focus:** Symmetry, aesthetics, visual appeal, comparison, external approval

- **Relationship to Pain:** Often ignored or glorified as necessary suffering for appearance

- **Training Motivation:** To sculpt an ideal form, gain attention, prove worth, control the uncontrollable

"I train to become admired, feared, lusted after, or envied. My body is the proof of my power."

🌀 Similarities: Where the Paths Intersect

Despite their contrast, these two approaches are not entirely at odds. In fact, they often begin to blur in the real lived experience of bodybuilders.

1. **Both Require Discipline and Devotion**

   Whether one is sculpting the body for divine embodiment or social validation, **intention, consistency, and effort** are required. The gym becomes a **sanctuary of transformation**—physical in both cases, spiritual in one.

2. **Both Recognize the Body as Transformable**

   The body is not static in either philosophy. It is **malleable**, shaped by thought, action, diet, energy, and belief. This implies a deep **interconnection between mind and matter**, a concept that can bridge both camps.

3. **Both Offer the Potential for Awakening**

   Ironically, even someone beginning with egoic or superficial motives may, over time, come to discover deeper truths through the process:

   - The discipline might lead to inner silence.

   - The mirror may become a tool for self-reflection beyond appearance.

   - Injury or burnout might catalyze a spiritual awakening or shift in purpose.

"The body that was once a mask can become a mirror."

◉ Integration: From Objectification to Sacred Embodiment

The true evolution of a bodybuilder may look like this:

1. **Starts with objectification:** Wanting to look like a superhero, be desired, prove worth.

2. **Moves through obsession:** Food, drugs, appearance, numbers, validation.

3. **Encounters the shadow:** Burnout, emptiness, disillusionment, injury, spiritual dryness.

4. **Discovers the vessel:** Begins listening, softening, understanding the body as sacred.

5. **Returns as integrated being:** Still trains, still sculpts—but now from love, reverence, devotion.

This shift doesn't mean abandoning aesthetics—it means **reclaiming aesthetics as divine art**, not as compensation for unhealed wounds.

🧘 Final Reflection: The Body as the Crossroads

In bodybuilding, the body is both **canvas and temple**—a place where vanity and virtue wrestle. The question is not which view is right, but **which consciousness is guiding your relationship to the body today**?

Is it fear or presence? Shame or reverence? Ego or soul?

When the body becomes a vessel for Spirit, every rep becomes prayer, every drop of sweat becomes offering. And in this shift, the bodybuilder becomes not just a sculptor of muscle, but a cultivator of consciousness.

❄ Spiritual Bodybuilding: A Path of Integration

📜 Definition

Spiritual Bodybuilding is not merely the pursuit of a physique—it is the conscious, intentional **integration of physical discipline with spiritual awakening**. It is using the gym, the diet, the pain, and the mirror as gateways into deeper **self-awareness, soul embodiment, and divine alignment**.

Integration: What Does It Really Mean?

To "integrate" means to unify what was once divided. In spiritual bodybuilding, this means:

Element	Fragmented State	Integrated State
Body	Object of desire or shame	Temple of awareness and sacred action
Mind	Tool for control or self-judgment	Ally in conscious evolution and clarity
Spirit	Disconnected or compartmentalized	Embodied, active within every rep, breath, and recovery
Training	Ego-driven, outcome obsessed	Ritual, meditation, pathway of self-refinement
Nutrition	Obsessive, joyless, controlling	Nourishing, intuitive, honoring digestion and rhythm
PEDs/Enhancement	Overuse, denial, addiction	Informed, intentional, with spiritual discernment
Suffering/Pain	Suppressed or glorified	Transmuted into meaning, resilience, and emotional access

Integration is not about perfection. It's about **embodying both shadow and light**, lifting through both heartbreak and gratitude, learning to **listen to the body** as a teacher rather than punish it into submission.

The Body as the Foundation of Awakening

In many spiritual traditions, the body has been bypassed in pursuit of "higher" consciousness. But in spiritual bodybuilding, we flip that script:

The body is not a hindrance to the soul—it is the soul's current home.

Through lifting, breathing, recovering, and fueling with intention, we are **literally building a temple that houses Spirit**. And with every disciplined act of self-respect, we say: "I am worthy of being here, of being whole, of being strong."

Bridging Masculine and Feminine Energies

Bodybuilding traditionally amplifies **masculine energy**: discipline, power, structure, achievement.

Spiritual integration invites the **feminine** back in:

- **Feeling over forcing**

- **Receptivity over rigidity**

- **Intuition alongside intention**

- **Flow with the form**

The **spiritual bodybuilder** becomes a living synthesis of **Shiva and Shakti**: focused, powerful, grounded—and also intuitive, compassionate, and deeply connected to life.

🌿 Performance Enhancement as Spiritual Responsibility

PEDs, peptides, supplements, even biohacking protocols—when divorced from spirit—become tools of ego, addiction, or illusion.

But when integrated into a **spirit-led practice**, they become:

- **Allies** in recovery

- **Catalysts** for healing

- **Mirrors** for inner imbalance

- **Gateways** to sacred self-mastery

This requires **radical honesty** and **intention**—asking not "How much can I take?" but "How deeply can I listen to what my body truly needs?"

🌐 Spiritual Bodybuilding as Initiation

This path is not unlike a **hero's journey** or **initiation rite**. It includes:

1. **Separation**: From the unconscious mainstream; deciding to forge your own way

2. **Descent**: Into shadow—addiction, disconnection, obsession, disillusionment

3. **Realization**: Pain leads to the truth: the body alone is not enough

4. **Healing**: Returning to presence, breath, spirit, support

5. **Return**: Emerging as an integrated being, with gifts to share

Each competition, each injury, each dietary phase or transformation becomes **alchemical**—turning raw experience into embodied wisdom.

Principles of the Spiritual Bodybuilder

1. **Train with presence.** Use each rep to feel, not escape.

2. **Eat with reverence.** Food is not just fuel—it is frequency.

3. **Supplement with integrity.** Ask if it honors the body's truth.

4. **Rest as devotion.** The nervous system is sacred.

5. **Embrace pain as a teacher.** Learn its language.

6. **Stay humble.** The body is temporary; the soul is not.

7. **Seek community.** Iron sharpens iron, but love softens stone.

Final Reflection: Becoming a Living Bridge

Spiritual bodybuilding is not just about muscles or macros.

It is a **return to wholeness**, a path where you become a bridge between:

- Earth and Sky

- Blood and Breath

- Sweat and Stillness

- Mirror and Meaning

To sculpt your body is to shape your devotion. To tame your ego is to free your essence. And to lift in love is to walk the divine path—one rep, one breath, one sacred step at a time.

It is very important to know and consistently remind yourself of what Bodybuilding means to you and what your WHY is for living this lifestyle. As you go through periods of time that require time, restriction, pushing your body and mind to the limits and possibly discovering new limits, coming back to the fundamental reason for doing it will keep you grounded in your truth and ensure that you keep yourself in check from getting sucked into the illusions that this lifestyle can pull you into.

Chapter 2: Muscle Hypertrophy as Spiritual Metaphor

Science of hypertrophy: microtrauma, recovery, supercompensation

✴ Hypertrophy: The Science of Growth Through Stress

🔬 The Biological Mechanism

At its core, **muscle hypertrophy** (muscle growth) is the result of:

1. **Mechanical tension** – created by resistance training, particularly under load and time under tension.

2. **Muscle damage** – microscopic tears (microtrauma) in muscle fibers.

3. **Metabolic stress** – accumulation of byproducts like lactate, causing cellular stress and hormonal responses.

These three factors signal the body that the current state of the muscle is **not enough** to handle the imposed demand.

This stress triggers a healing response, and in the process of repairing itself, the muscle becomes **bigger, stronger, and more resilient**—this is **supercompensation**.

⊟ The Cycle of Adaptation

The hypertrophic process unfolds in a spiritual rhythm:

Stage	Scientific Term	Spiritual Parallel
Challenge	Microtrauma	Initiation / Ego Death
Surrender & Rest	Recovery	Integration / Stillness
Rebirth	Supercompensation	Transcendence / Renewal

Each training session is a ritual in **controlled breakdown**—where the body willingly enters stress in order to evolve. But without recovery, there is no growth. And without intention, there is no meaning.

🜊 The Spiritual Alchemy of Hypertrophy

The physical act of tearing muscle tissue is a **spiritual metaphor**: in order to grow, we must first be **broken open**.

💧 Microtrauma as Initiation

- In hypertrophy, **microtrauma** is essential. Without tension, there is no adaptation.

- Spiritually, we encounter "microtrauma" in our daily lives: heartbreaks, setbacks, disillusionment, failures.

- Each "tear" to our identity or comfort zone becomes an opportunity for **evolution**, if we allow ourselves to feel and heal.

The sacred paradox: **What wounds you can also awaken you.**

Recovery as Sacred Integration

- True growth doesn't happen during training—it happens during **rest, sleep**, and **deep nourishment**.

- Spiritually, this reflects the value of **meditation**, **inner stillness**, and **emotional digestion**.

- Just as the nervous system requires downregulation to repair tissues, the **soul requires silence to reweave itself**.

Overtraining is not strength—it's **spiritual bypassing through action**.

Supercompensation as Ascension

- Once the muscle recovers, it rebounds to a level **beyond its former state**.

- This is **transcendence through experience**: the "you" that lifts today is not the same "you" who recovers tomorrow.

- It echoes the **death and rebirth cycles** found in initiatory rites, mythology, and alchemical transformation.

Anabolic Signaling: The Voice of Growth

The body communicates its readiness to grow through hormonal messengers:

- **mTOR pathway activation** – signals protein synthesis

- **Testosterone, GH, IGF-1** – promote tissue repair and hypertrophy

- **Cortisol** – catabolic when chronic, but essential in acute training stress

- **Myokines** – muscle-released peptides that signal adaptation and even affect **brain function** and **emotion**

These molecules aren't just chemicals—they're **sacred messengers of evolution**.

Spiritual bodybuilding sees this as **inner alchemy**: your training is not just building muscle—it's awakening the endocrine and nervous systems as a **feedback loop with your higher self**.

✦ Key Spiritual Principles of Hypertrophy

1. **Tension is transformation in disguise.**

- Don't avoid the pain—learn its purpose.

2. **Recovery is sacred.**

- True strength is in how well you heal, not just how hard you train.

3. **Growth requires cycles.**

- Embrace your seasons: push, pause, repair, ascend.

4. **Intentionality rewires physiology.**

- Training with presence enhances neural recruitment, hormonal output, and energetic imprinting.

5. **The body is your sacred forge.**

- Every rep is a prayer. Every set, a sacred contract with the future version of you.

🧘 Practical Integration Practices

To truly embody the spiritual path of hypertrophy:

- **Begin each training session with breathwork or intention setting.**

- **Finish each workout in stillness, gratitude, or light stretching.**

- **Cycle your training for energetic balance:** heavy lifting → deload → mobility/yoga → return to strength.

- **Use journaling after intense phases** to process emotional shifts.

- **Honor sleep, digestion, and emotional states** as essential parts of muscle growth.

- **Ask: What part of me is growing beyond just the muscle?**

Closing Thought

Hypertrophy is more than adaptation—it's **remembrance**.

In tearing down what we were, we become what we are destined to be—not just physically, but energetically. The muscle is the metaphor. The real growth is within.

Discipline, Consistency, and Resistance: Sacred Teachers of the Soul

In the iron temple of bodybuilding, weights are not just tools of the trade—they are **mirrors of the soul**. Beneath every rep, every drop of sweat, and every early morning alarm lies a trio of hidden initiators: **discipline, consistency, and resistance**. These are not just habits—they are **spiritual technologies** that refine the character and forge the deeper self.

1. Discipline: The Sword That Cuts Through Chaos

Discipline is not punishment. It is the sacred choice to align with one's **higher self**, moment by moment.

In a world addicted to distraction and instant gratification, discipline teaches us to delay the lesser reward for the **greater becoming**. It requires saying no to the lower impulses—not out of shame, but out of reverence for the person we are becoming.

Spiritually, discipline is the fire of **devotion**—a daily affirmation that our body is a temple and our time, a gift.

Every time we show up—tired, uncertain, uninspired—we transmute resistance into reverence. Discipline teaches **patience**, because results are slow. And it teaches **humility**, because it reminds us we are not entitled to transformation without effort.

2. Consistency: The Drumbeat of Becoming

Where discipline is the sword, **consistency is the heartbeat**.

Anyone can be motivated for a week. But **consistency is the surrender to process**. It humbles the ego that craves quick results and instant aesthetics. It trains us to look beyond surface-level gratification and invest in the long game—the **unseen cultivation of spirit over time**.

Every act of consistency is a prayer, a vote cast for who we desire to become.

In bodybuilding, progress may be invisible for weeks, even months. But the soul knows. It's in the subtle alignment of your values with your actions. Consistency softens our need to control the outcome and strengthens our trust in divine timing. We learn that mastery is not a destination—it is a rhythm.

3. Resistance: The Invisible Teacher

Without resistance, there is no growth. This is true for muscle tissue—and for the soul.

The barbell gets heavier. Life gets more complicated. Motivation fades. These are not obstacles—they are **initiations**. Resistance teaches us to **respect the process**. It reveals our edges, our limitations, our shadows. And in doing so, it gives us the gift of **humility**.

In the gym and in life, resistance whispers, "You are not yet who you could be."

Through resistance, we encounter our impatience, our ego, our fears. But when we meet it with presence and breath, it becomes a teacher—not a tormentor.

The Spiritual Alchemy of Patience and Humility

- **Patience** is the fruit of enduring cycles without forcing the outcome. It teaches **trust** in the unseen, and reverence for divine timing.

- **Humility** is born when we realize that effort alone does not guarantee outcome. It softens our arrogance and opens us to **grace**—to learning, to failure, and to surrender.

Bodybuilding without patience becomes obsession.

Bodybuilding without humility becomes narcissism.

But with both, it becomes **spiritual initiation**—a union of body, mind, and soul.

Final Reflection

Discipline, consistency, and resistance are the **unsung gurus** of the spiritual bodybuilder. They do not shout; they whisper. They do not entertain; they transform. And if we are willing to be students, they will not only sculpt our bodies—they will reveal our essence.

Chapter 3: Weight Training as Meditation

When most people enter the gym, they carry noise with them: the noise of daily stress, the noise of comparison, the noise of ego. They load the barbell as if it will silence that noise through sheer force, but more often it amplifies it. True transformation begins when the gym is no longer just a place to sculpt the body, but a place to still the mind and deepen the spirit. Weight training, approached with reverence and awareness, becomes meditation in motion.

Presence in the Lift

Meditation begins with presence, and so does lifting. Each rep is a call to return to the body, to feel the texture of the bar in your hands, the ground beneath your feet, and the subtle shifts of balance as weight moves through you. Presence sharpens awareness. In this state, distraction dissolves, and what remains is the living dialogue between muscle, breath, and mind.

Biochemically, presence reduces the scatter of cortisol-driven reactivity. It shifts training out of anxious fight-or-flight and into a state of flow where parasympathetic calm meets sympathetic strength. Spiritually, presence is the gateway — the doorway to turn effort into prayer.

Breath as the Guide

Every rep is a breath cycle. Inhale to prepare, exhale to release. The rhythm of respiration synchronizes effort and awareness. Breath anchors the nervous system and regulates the Bohr effect — ensuring oxygen reaches tissues efficiently, fueling both strength and clarity.

When you align breath with movement, lifting transcends exertion. It becomes pranayama with iron: the barbell becomes a tool to harness life-force, to unify body and spirit through breath.

Intention Over Ego

Ego wants more: more weight, more plates, more validation. But meditation asks: why? Lifting with intention replaces the pursuit of external approval with inner dialogue. Numbers matter less than alignment. The bar is no longer a rival but a teacher.

Physically, this reduces injury risk. Emotionally, it frees you from the tyranny of comparison. Spiritually, it transforms training into ritual — intention as offering, not performance.

Mind–Muscle Connection as Mantra

Just as meditation uses mantras to focus awareness, weight training uses contraction. The sensation of a muscle shortening, fibers aligning under tension, becomes the mantra of the body. Each repetition is a recitation, a return to the present moment.

Neurologically, this practice deepens motor unit recruitment, sharpening performance. Emotionally, it develops trust in the body. Spiritually, it is devotion: every rep is prayer, every contraction a bead on the rosary of discipline.

Controlled Tempo as Mind Control

The impatient lifter thrashes through reps, but the mindful lifter moves with deliberate tempo. Slowness cultivates mastery. Controlling time under tension is controlling mind under stress.

Biochemically, slower tempo reduces adrenaline spikes and teaches cortisol to stay balanced. Emotionally, it forges patience. Spiritually, it is the art of living deliberately, of refusing to be rushed by the ego's hunger for more.

Tension as Energy Awareness

Tension is not just mechanical — it is energetic. Fascia, breath, and intention form pathways for life-force to flow. Lifting teaches us where energy stagnates: the tight hips storing grief, the shoulders carrying unspoken burdens.

By engaging these points with awareness, the lifter becomes an energy worker. Biochemically, tension reflects energy demand and lactate signaling. Spiritually, it is awareness of prana, chi, the currents of subtle energy that animate the body.

Failure as Surrender

To train to failure is to confront surrender. Muscles tremble, breath quickens, the weight refuses to move. In this moment, ego dies. You are forced to release control, to feel vulnerability without collapse.

Physically, failure is hormesis — breakdown leading to adaptation. Emotionally, it teaches humility. Spiritually, it mirrors the mystical experience: the death of self, the birth of transformation.

Rest as Reflection

In meditation, the silence between mantras is as sacred as the chant itself. In lifting, rest between sets is reflection. It is the integration of stress and release.

Physiologically, recovery is where growth occurs — protein synthesis, GH release, glycogen replenishment. Emotionally, it is pause and assimilation. Spiritually, it is the sacred gap, the silence between the notes of a song.

Consistency as Discipline of Spirit

Meditation is not about one session but about daily return. Weight training, too, rewards consistency. Each session, each cycle, each year builds not only muscle but character. Discipline is the slow weaving of devotion into the fabric of life.

Biochemically, consistent training reinforces circadian rhythm and stabilizes hormones. Emotionally, it grounds you in structure. Spiritually, it is devotion in action: returning to the temple, to the altar of the barbell.

Strength as Stillness Embodied

At its highest level, strength is not aggression — it is serenity under load. True strength is not how much you can thrash, but how still you can remain in the storm of resistance.

Physically, it is balanced muscle and nervous system integration. Biochemically, it is mitochondrial resilience. Emotionally, it is confidence without arrogance. Spiritually, it is equanimity: the ability to carry weight without being weighed down.

Integration: The Barbell as Prayer Bead

Weight training as meditation is not about technique alone. It is about changing the quality of awareness we bring into the gym. When we lift with presence, breath, intention, and surrender, the barbell becomes more than iron. It becomes a prayer bead, each rep a mantra, each set a meditation.

The body grows, yes — but so do patience, clarity, and connection. In this alchemy of muscle and mindfulness, bodybuilding transcends its outer shell and becomes spiritual practice. Strength becomes stillness, and the gym becomes temple.

Chapter 4: The Alchemy and Illusion of Performance Enhancement

A. Performance Enhancing Drugs (PEDs) Overview

Chronic supra-physiological levels of testosterone—meaning levels consistently above the natural biological range—can have significant impacts not only on the body and psyche, but also on the subtler layers of consciousness often referred to in spiritual or energetic frameworks.

Here's a breakdown of potential **spiritual implications** through various lenses:

1. Energetic and Chakra System View

In many spiritual traditions, hormonal states are deeply tied to **chakra function** and **energy flow**.

- **Excessive testosterone** tends to overstimulate the **solar plexus (Manipura)** and **root (Muladhara)** chakras.

- This can result in an **overemphasis on willpower, dominance, competition, sex, aggression**, and **physicality**, potentially leading to imbalance.

- When not balanced by the **heart (Anahata)** and **third eye (Ajna)** chakras, this may create a disconnect from empathy, intuition, and spiritual insight.

⊚ **Spiritual consequence**: A soul may become *over-anchored* in the material realm—fixated on control, strength, and external validation—limiting its capacity for higher transcendence, surrender, or unity consciousness.

2. Masculine Archetype Distortion

Testosterone amplifies traits associated with the **divine masculine**—clarity, decisiveness, protection, and drive.

- In chronic excess, these can become **distorted into shadow forms**: tyranny instead of leadership, hypersexuality instead of sacred union, domination instead of grounded presence.

- This distortion can manifest in the psyche as spiritual pride, spiritual bypassing, or an unwillingness to be vulnerable or humble before mystery.

 Spiritual consequence: The journey inward may be blocked by an inflated ego or an armored identity that fears surrender, softness, and the unknown.

3. Imbalance of Yin and Yang

In Taoist philosophy, testosterone correlates with **Yang** energy—active, fiery, outward, forceful.

- A surplus of Yang without adequate **Yin** (receptivity, stillness, inwardness) can create a kind of **spiritual burnout**, leading to restlessness, insomnia, inability to meditate, or an aversion to emotional depth.

- It can also disturb the flow of **Qi** (life force), leading to energetic rigidity or stagnation.

 Spiritual consequence: The person may become disconnected from the feminine aspect of divinity, intuition, or the womb-like stillness from which all true spiritual insights arise.

🧬 4. Karma and Soul Lessons

On a soul level, chronic excess testosterone may be part of a karmic journey involving the **exploration of power, drive, sexuality, and identity**.

- The soul may have chosen a path to master these forces—not by denying them, but by learning to **wield them with love, consciousness, and sacred intention**.

- Alternatively, it could represent an **avoidance of deeper emotional wounds**, where testosterone becomes a shield against vulnerability.

🧘 **Spiritual opportunity**: To integrate primal power with divine compassion— becoming a "warrior of the heart" rather than a force of unchecked will.

🧘 5. Detachment from Spirit or Soul Guidance

In some individuals, heightened testosterone can create a kind of **energetic "loudness"** that drowns out the quieter voice of inner guidance, ancestors, or higher self.

- Meditation becomes harder, subtle perceptions are muted, and life becomes oriented around conquest, stimulation, and performance.

🧠 **Spiritual consequence**: A loss of subtlety in one's perception of Spirit; a forgetting of why we incarnated in the first place.

🕊️ Healing and Balance

To restore spiritual harmony, one might:

- Cultivate **yin practices**: breathwork, gentle yoga, stillness, deep listening.

- Balance physical strength with **emotional vulnerability and shadow work**.

- Engage in **plant medicine**, ritual, or body-based spirituality to reintegrate disowned parts of the self.

- Reflect on **what drives the need for more**—what wound is masked by power, sex, or control?

Let's explore the **spiritual implications of chronically low testosterone, which will inevitably happen after prolonged supra-physiological dosing of Testosterone,** through a multidimensional lens:

1. Energetic and Chakra System View

Low testosterone often corresponds with **deficient energy in the root (Muladhara)** and **solar plexus (Manipura)** chakras—those that govern:

- Grounding and safety (root)

- Willpower, identity, and action (solar plexus)

- When these centers are underactive:

- A person may feel **ungrounded, passive, indecisive**, or **lacking in life-force drive**.

- The physical world may feel **unsafe or overwhelming**, and the ability to manifest intentions into action may be hindered.

Spiritual implication: There can be a tendency to retreat from embodiment—to live more in the upper chakras or in the astral/spiritual realms—losing touch with earthly purpose or material participation.

2. Wounding Around the Masculine

Testosterone is a physical expression of **masculine life force**, and chronic low levels can point to **spiritual wounding related to the masculine archetype.**

This might show up as:

- Fear of asserting oneself

- Rejection of masculine energy due to trauma (e.g., abusive father figures, war, toxic patriarchy)

- A karmic pattern of suppressing aggression, anger, or sexual energy out of guilt, shame, or spiritual over-identification with peace/passivity

⚖️ **Spiritual implication**: The soul may be working through lifetimes of **disempowerment or aversion to power**, choosing to experience humility, gentleness, or even helplessness as a counterbalance.

🪶 3. Yin Over-expression and Shadow Feminine

Just as high testosterone reflects overactive **Yang**, low testosterone often represents an **over-dominance of Yin**—receptivity, stillness, softness—but sometimes to the point of disempowerment or collapse.

It may bring:

- Emotional hypersensitivity

- Lack of boundaries

- Difficulty in protecting or asserting the self

- Tendency to live in fantasy or dissociation

🪶 **Spiritual implication**: The person may have strong intuitive or psychic gifts but struggles to **anchor them into form** or act upon their visions. They may become spiritually porous, vulnerable to energetic interference, or emotionally overwhelmed.

4. An Invitation to Rebuild Authentic Power

Low testosterone can be seen as an **initiation into a different kind of strength**—not physical or sexual dominance, but **inner fortitude**, clarity, and calm presence.

It asks:

- What does it mean to be powerful *without force*?

- How can I show up with dignity, even when I feel "less than"?

- Can I learn to act from alignment, not adrenaline?

Spiritual opportunity: To **redefine masculinity** or inner power on your own terms—reclaiming sacred action, sacred anger, and grounded sexuality without the distortions of dominance or ego.

5. Suppressed Kundalini or Life Force Energy

Testosterone is closely linked to **libido**, which in many traditions is seen as a **manifestation of kundalini energy**—creative, erotic, and divine.

Low testosterone may reflect a **block in the flow of this life force**, especially if there's shame, trauma, or repression around sexuality or primal instinct.

Spiritual implication: The soul may be calling for a **reawakening of the serpent energy**—not just for sexual vitality, but as a path to spiritual transformation, embodiment, and self-realization.

Pathways to Integration and Healing

Here are spiritual and energetic ways to work with low testosterone as a growth catalyst:

- **Embodiment practices**: strength training, qigong, primal movement, cold exposure—done with spiritual awareness, not ego.

- **Shadow work around masculinity**: Explore your lineage, father wounds, ancestral karma, or vows (e.g., vows of celibacy, powerlessness).

- **Tantric or sexual energy work**: Cultivating life-force through breath, self-touch, connection to the Earth and your own sacred sensuality.

- **Earth-rooted spirituality**: Work with root chakra stones (hematite, garnet), grounding herbs (ashwagandha, maca), and nature immersion.

💜 Most of all, this imbalance often invites the **reconciliation of the Divine Feminine and Divine Masculine within**—not in competition, but in sacred partnership.

B. Chronic HGH, Thyroid & Insulin Abuse: Spiritual Implications

HGH: unnatural acceleration of growth = spiritual bypassing of life cycles

HGH and the Unnatural Acceleration of Growth: The Cost of Skipping Sacred Cycles

1. Biochemical Acceleration: The Metabolic Cost of Skipping Time

Human Growth Hormone (HGH) is secreted by the anterior pituitary gland and is integral to:

- **Tissue repair**

- **Muscle growth**

- **Cell regeneration**

- **Bone density**

- **Fat metabolism**

Endogenously, HGH pulses during sleep, fasting, and intense exercise, aligning with **natural rhythms of growth, recovery, and maturation**.

When we supplement HGH exogenously—especially in supra-physiological doses— we **override this wisdom**, forcing the body into a constant **anabolic, growth-driven state** that would not otherwise occur.

Biochemical Consequences:

- **IGF-1 Overexpression**: HGH boosts **Insulin-like Growth Factor 1**, which stimulates cell proliferation but may increase cancer risk if unregulated.

- **Insulin Resistance**: HGH antagonizes insulin. Chronic elevation often leads to hyperglycemia and **pre-diabetic conditions**.

- **Joint and Organ Overgrowth**: Not just muscle grows. **Cartilage, soft tissue, heart, and even intestines** can enlarge, risking long-term complications.

- **Reduced Endogenous Production**: Supplementation suppresses natural pituitary output, making the user dependent.

Summary: Biochemically, HGH creates an **artificial state of growth** that stresses the endocrine system and can distort the body's intended equilibrium.

2. Physical Overreach: Building What the Soul Hasn't Earned

Physically, HGH enables rapid transformations—**faster muscle gain, fat loss, tissue healing, and skin rejuvenation**. On the surface, it appears miraculous.

But nature's cycles are **slow for a reason**. Each phase—**breakdown, rest, repair, renewal**—has spiritual intelligence embedded within it. When we rush growth, we:

- Bypass the lessons of limitation.

- Avoid the humility of time and patience.

- Build bodies that **look ready** but lack the **energetic foundation** to sustain that readiness.

This manifests as:

- Fragile strength

- External overdevelopment with internal underdevelopment

- A disconnect between physical power and emotional/spiritual maturity

A body forged by unnatural growth can become a false temple—impressive, yet uninhabited.

3. Emotional Dislocation: The Insecurity Beneath the Enhancement

HGH use is often driven not by confidence, but **insecurity disguised as ambition**:

- Fear of aging

- Fear of not being "enough"

- Fear of being left behind in a competitive world

Because HGH provides **immediate feedback** (rapid results), it becomes addictive— reinforcing the cycle of:

"I must be better. I must be younger. I must be more."

This fast-forward approach to improvement **disconnects the user from the emotional growth that comes from struggle**, setbacks, and surrender.

Common emotional outcomes include:

- **Heightened body dysmorphia**

- **Impatience and irritability**

- **Attachment to external validation**

- **Difficulty resting or doing less**

4. Spiritual Bypassing: Escaping the Sacred Phases of the Human Journey

Spiritually, HGH presents a powerful metaphor: **amplify growth without embracing the seasons that precede it**.

Nature teaches us that:

- **Winter** (rest/death) precedes **Spring** (rebirth).

- **Stillness** precedes **transformation**.

- **Crisis** precedes **clarity**.

When HGH is used to bypass these cycles, we:

- **Escape the death-rebirth archetype**, robbing ourselves of wisdom.

- **Disown our aging process**, cutting off our access to elder consciousness.

- **Inhabit a shell of perpetual youth**, but lose the initiatory rites that would deepen our soul.

The user remains in "Spring," endlessly blooming without ever surrendering to the cycles of death and renewal.

This is **spiritual bypassing**: using enhancement to escape the sacred discomfort that refines character, insight, and depth.

The Alternative: Slow Growth as Sacred Growth

Not all enhancement is wrong. But sacred enhancement requires:

- **Deep self-honesty** about motives

- **Alignment with nature's wisdom** (i.e., respecting rest, rhythm, and integration)

- **Maturity to delay gratification** for deeper transformation

The spiritual bodybuilder understands:

- **The muscle isn't the point—it's the mirror.**

- **Growth is earned, not injected.**

- **A temple cannot be rushed—it must be lived into.**

Conclusion: When Growth Becomes Hollow

Taking HGH to skip phases of life is not just a biochemical shortcut—it is a **philosophical and spiritual fracture**. It creates a body that **appears evolved but isn't rooted in earned truth**.

To truly grow is to integrate:

- **Tension with release**

- **Youth with age**

- **Masculine doing with feminine being**

- **Power with wisdom**

When we honor the **seasons of becoming**, we grow a body that is not just strong— but sacred.

Thyroid Hormones in Performance Enhancement

In bodybuilding and athletic performance, synthetic thyroid hormones—primarily **T3 (liothyronine)** and sometimes **T4 (levothyroxine)**—are often used to increase metabolic rate and accelerate fat loss. While this can lead to a leaner physique in the short term, the implications on **biochemistry, physiology, and spiritual integrity** are profound when misused.

Biochemical & Physiological Effects

Short-Term Effects

- **Increased Basal Metabolic Rate (BMR):** T3 upregulates the mitochondria, increasing cellular respiration and calorie burn.

- **Fat Loss Acceleration:** Lipolysis is enhanced, especially when combined with calorie deficits and stimulants.

- **Energy Boost (Transient):** The user may feel energized, mentally sharp, and hyper-motivated initially.

- **Muscle Catabolism:** T3 is catabolic; without careful dosing and nutrition, it often burns muscle tissue along with fat.

- **Disrupted Hormonal Signaling:** Supplementing T3/T4 suppresses the hypothalamic-pituitary-thyroid (HPT) axis, shutting down natural thyroid production.

Long-Term Effects

- **Thyroid Suppression:** Chronic use can permanently downregulate endogenous thyroid function, requiring lifelong replacement therapy.

- **Adrenal Fatigue:** The artificially elevated metabolism strains the adrenals, often leading to cortisol dysregulation, anxiety, and burnout.

- **Cardiovascular Stress:** Long-term elevated thyroid activity increases heart rate, blood pressure, and arrhythmia risk.

- **Nutrient Deficiencies:** T3 depletes magnesium, zinc, selenium, and B vitamins—cofactors needed for thyroid and metabolic health.

- **Mitochondrial Damage:** Prolonged overstimulation of mitochondria can lead to oxidative stress and cellular dysfunction.

Spiritual Implications

Thyroid function is deeply tied to **expression, alignment, and authenticity**—it governs the **throat chakra** (Vishuddha), which is the energetic center of **truth, communication, and willpower**. When we chemically override this center for aesthetic or performance gains, there are spiritual consequences:

1. Disharmony with Inner Rhythms

Artificial stimulation of metabolism often disconnects us from our natural energetic cycles. This creates a state of **chronic inner pressure**, where the body is forced to "do" rather than "be." We lose the ability to hear the whispers of the soul because we're chasing the noise of the ego.

2. Silencing the Voice of the Self

The thyroid governs **voice and expression**. Chronic T3 use can lead to a paradox where external image is amplified, but internal authenticity is suppressed. One may feel increasingly alienated from their true motivations, trapped in a loop of **performance-based identity**.

3. Loss of Intuition

Pushing the body out of its natural hormonal rhythm dampens somatic intelligence. Hunger, fatigue, rest, and stillness become "problems to fix," not signals to honor. Over time, this leads to **disembodiment**, spiritual disorientation, and emotional instability.

4. Karma of Manipulation

From a metaphysical lens, using thyroid hormones as a shortcut to leanness may represent a karmic pattern of **forcing outcomes rather than allowing transformation**. It becomes a symbolic act of distrusting the divine timing of the body and soul's journey.

When, If Ever, Is It Appropriate?

In rare cases, **low-dose thyroid support** (e.g., for subclinical hypothyroidism) may be a legitimate tool for wellness or competition prep under clinical guidance. In these contexts, it must be used with:

- **Medical supervision**

- **Proper lab tracking** (TSH, FT3, FT4, rT3)

- **Minimum effective dose**

- **Strict cycling and tapering**

- **Emotional grounding and spiritual discernment**

Reintegration and Healing After Thyroid Use

If someone has misused thyroid hormones, recovery is possible:

Biochemical Protocols

- Re-establish HPT axis function with adaptogens (e.g., ashwagandha, rhodiola), selenium, iodine (with caution), zinc, and B-complex.

- Support liver and gut health (where T4 converts to T3).

- Use **cold exposure and breathwork** to regulate the endocrine system naturally.

Spiritual Practices

- **Throat chakra clearing** through chanting, journaling, honest conversation, and singing.

- **Return to presence:** meditation, stillness, nature immersion.

- **Release of ego-based goals**: reconnect with purpose and joy rather than outcomes.

Conclusion: The Body as Oracle, Not Object

Enhancing the body should be a celebration of its sacred design, not a denial of its wisdom. When we override our endocrine system for aesthetics, we risk silencing the soul. But when we learn to **listen, support, and evolve**—the body becomes a living prayer, not a performance.

- **Insulin**: manipulates life's energy currency (glucose) = playing god with fuel

The Alchemy of Insulin: Weaponizing the Hormone of Life

Insulin is one of the most **potent and paradoxical** hormones in the human body. It is both the key to life and, when misused, a doorway to destruction.

In the world of bodybuilding, insulin is often used to shuttle nutrients more efficiently—especially glucose and amino acids—into the muscle cell, creating **faster recovery, fuller muscle bellies, and dramatic mass gain**.

But behind the anabolic utility lies a much deeper **spiritual risk**: the distortion of nature's rhythm, emotional avoidance, and the potential erosion of intuitive intelligence in the body.

1. Biochemical Mechanics: Harnessing the Anabolic Key

Insulin is secreted by the pancreas in response to elevated blood glucose levels. Its core functions:

- Shuttles **glucose** into cells for energy or storage (as glycogen or fat)

- Stimulates **amino acid** uptake and **protein synthesis**

- Inhibits **lipolysis** (fat burning)

- Regulates nutrient partitioning and metabolic balance

When used pharmacologically, insulin:

- Dramatically **increases nutrient uptake**, particularly post-training

- Enhances **glycogen storage** and intracellular hydration (which makes muscles appear bigger)

- Can synergize with **growth hormone and anabolic steroids** to amplify hypertrophy

However, insulin is also **highly dangerous** if mismanaged:

- Risk of **hypoglycemia** (low blood sugar), which can lead to dizziness, coma, or death

- **Rebound fat gain** from excess carbohydrate intake

- Suppression of **endogenous insulin sensitivity** if chronically abused

What begins as anabolic science can quickly become metabolic chaos.

2. Physical Impact: Fullness Without Function

On the surface, insulin use can create:

- **Rounder, fuller muscles**

- **Rapid weight gain**

- **Improved post-workout recovery**

But this comes with trade-offs:

- Many users accumulate **visceral fat** alongside muscle

- The muscle gained can feel **puffy, watery, or unstable**—not dense, dry, or truly functional

- Long-term use can lead to **insulin resistance**, metabolic syndrome, and even Type 2 diabetes

The body begins to prioritize **appearance over efficiency**—it becomes a visual illusion of power, rather than an integrated engine of performance.

It's the difference between a balloon and a brick: both may be the same size, but only one carries true weight.

3. Emotional Drivers: Chasing Fullness to Avoid Emptiness

The psychological and emotional motivators behind insulin use often trace back to:

- **Body dysmorphia**: Never feeling big or full enough

- **Fear of stagnation**: Wanting faster progress regardless of cost

- **Impatience and control issues**: Forcing growth instead of earning it

Insulin provides **instant gratification**—more size, more pump, more "presence." But it **masks rather than heals** the deeper voids many athletes carry:

- The need for approval

- The fear of disappearing without size

- The false belief that worth is measured in inches and vascularity

Over time, insulin becomes not just a physical tool—but a **psychological crutch**.

4. Spiritual Consequences: Distorting Nature's Flow

Insulin, when respected, is the **essence of nourishment**. It is the energetic bridge between sustenance and structure. It turns food into form.

When manipulated aggressively, insulin becomes a **tool of bypass and distortion**:

- It shortcuts growth

- It overrides hunger and satiety signals

- It severs the body's **natural relationship with food, rhythm, and rest**

From a spiritual perspective, insulin misuse reflects:

- **A refusal to trust the timeline of transformation**

- **An ego-driven impulse to "fill the void" without understanding it**

- **A misalignment between outer growth and inner evolution**

True muscle is sacred architecture, built slowly with intention and struggle. Insulin abuse erects a false temple—visually impressive, but spiritually vacant.

In metaphysical terms, insulin governs **sacred receptivity**—how we absorb, assimilate, and store the life force. When used artificially, we train the body to **receive unnaturally**, and over time this may mirror spiritual states of:

- Greed

- Gluttony

- Overconsumption

- Lack of discernment

5. The Danger of Addiction to Fullness

A major trap with insulin is the **emotional addiction to the pump**:

- Post-injection, nutrient-loaded muscles swell dramatically

- Over time, this becomes a **neurochemical high**—not unlike a drug rush

- Coming off insulin can feel like deflation, leading to depressive dips or anxiety

This pattern reinforces **external identity attachment**:

- "I am what I look like."

- "I must maintain fullness or I'll lose relevance."

- "I need to stay huge or I won't love myself."

The soul becomes a slave to the body's illusion.

6. A Conscious Relationship to Insulin

If one were to use insulin later in life with full awareness, it must come with:

- **Deep education** about carb timing, glycemic index, and insulin sensitivity

- **Metabolic markers monitoring** (fasting glucose, HbA1c, insulin levels)

- **Post-cycle recovery plans**, including berberine, chromium, bitter melon, and fasting protocols

- An honest **emotional and spiritual check-in**:

  - *Why am I using this?*

  - *What part of me believes I need to accelerate growth this way?*

  - *Am I chasing something I could cultivate more slowly with love and presence?*

Conclusion: Don't Confuse Fullness with Wholeness

Insulin is not inherently evil. It is a sacred hormone—the alchemist of fuel into form.

But when used recklessly, it teaches us a hard truth:

You can force the body to grow, but not the soul.

Spiritual bodybuilding means honoring **timing**, **balance**, and **truth**. It means building a body that can hold more light, not just more glycogen. It means understanding that **being full is not the same as being fulfilled.**

The Final substance of Note, and very important to recognize within this Generation, is the use and abuse of Trenbolone.

TREN: THE DARK ALCHEMY OF PERFORMANCE

Trenbolone is often called the "King of Steroids"—and not without reason. It is a compound of **extreme potency**, capable of transforming a physique in weeks, yet carrying with it a **shadow frequency** that can be devastating to mind, body, and spirit.

To use Tren is to dance with fire. The muscle gains are real—but so is the madness.

1. Biochemical Profile: The Chemistry of Command

Trenbolone is a 19-nor anabolic steroid, derived from nandrolone, with an **anabolic-androgenic ratio** estimated at **500:500** (compared to testosterone's 100:100). This makes it one of the most **anabolically and androgenically intense compounds** in existence.

<u>Key Biochemical Effects:</u>

- **Increased nitrogen retention** → enhanced muscle protein synthesis

- **Increased red blood cell count** → more oxygen transport, more endurance

- **Enhanced IGF-1 expression** → synergizes with growth factors for hypertrophy

- **Suppressed glucocorticoids** → anti-catabolic effect, reducing muscle breakdown

<u>But it also:</u>

- **Shuts down natural testosterone production** almost immediately

- **Raises prolactin levels**, causing mood swings and potential gyno

- **Elevates cortisol post-cycle**, risking adrenal disruption and HPA-axis damage

- **Disrupts dopamine/serotonin signaling**, impairing emotional regulation

Tren hijacks the body's chemistry, weaponizing it for anabolic warfare—while draining its reservoirs of natural balance.

2. Physical Effects: A Body Like Stone—But At What Cost?

Positive (Short-Term) Effects:

- Rapid, dry, dense muscle gain

- Extreme vascularity and hardness

- Accelerated fat loss (powerful nutrient partitioning)

- Enhanced aggression and drive during training

<u>Negative (Short-Term) Effects:</u>

- **"Tren Cough"** from oil-based injection entering bloodstream

- **Insomnia**, often described as "wired but tired"

- **Night sweats**, thermogenic side effects from metabolic ramping

- **Cardiovascular stress**, including elevated BP and lipid derangement

<u>Long-Term Consequences:</u>

- **Heart enlargement and fibrosis**, due to chronic high blood pressure and cardiac strain

- **Neurotoxicity**, with altered dopamine and GABA signaling

- **Kidney and liver toxicity**, particularly from Trenbolone acetate

- **Loss of fertility and permanent HPTA suppression**

Tren makes you look like a god—and feel like a ghost.

3. Emotional and Psychological Impact: The Mind in Conflict

Common psychological symptoms:

- **Severe mood swings**

- **Paranoia, anxiety, irritability**

- **Loss of emotional bandwidth**

- **Increased aggressive tendencies**

- **Obsessive thought patterns and body dysmorphia**

Many users report feeling **cut off from their heart space**—operating purely from the head, or worse, the ego.

On Tren, some men report being emotionally numb, others feel hyper-sensitive and reactive. Either way, it becomes difficult to **regulate inner states**, leading to a fractured sense of identity.

Relationships suffer. Intimacy suffers. Authentic expression becomes hard to access.

The emotional cost of Tren is not spoken about enough—but it is often the most devastating.

4. Spiritual Implications: Ego Ascending, Spirit Descending

Tren represents **an extreme expression of yang energy**—control, force, dominance, separation.

It empowers the shadow masculine:

- Domination over flow

- Hyper-competitiveness

- Suppression of vulnerability

- Sacrifice of balance for victory

Tren and Spiritual Bypassing:

By accelerating results beyond what's naturally sustainable, Tren encourages the user to:

- **Avoid inner work**

- **Attach to outer identity**

- **Seek validation through form alone**

- **Neglect cycles of rest, recovery, and reflection**

There is no time to listen to the body. Only time to conquer it.

Tren bypasses the organic timeline of the soul. It creates hypertrophy without humility—size without stillness. It elevates the body and suppresses the spirit.

Energetic Consequences:
- Aura becomes **dense, rigid, forceful**

- Heart space often closes, compassion narrows

- Chakras become unbalanced—particularly **solar plexus** (power), **root** (survival), and **third eye** (intuition)

- Connection to the divine weakens in favor of **ego inflation and separation consciousness**

5. Shadow Patterns of Use

Tren is often used during cutting or competition preps, but many abuse it year-round due to its addicting visual results. This creates:

- **Chronically elevated stress hormones**

- **Neurochemical dependency on "rage" and intensity**

- A pattern of **self-punishment disguised as discipline**

It becomes a **spiritual possession** of sorts—where the user becomes controlled by the compound.

6. Recovery and Reconciliation

Coming off Tren can feel like **emotional death**:

- Crashes in testosterone and dopamine

- Feelings of emptiness, weakness, depression

- In some cases, suicidal ideation

This is the soul calling for **re-integration**.

If Tren has been used, recovery must be:

- **Physiological**: PCT, adrenal/hepatic/kidney support, balanced training

- **Psychological**: Therapy, integration coaching, journaling, reconnecting to purpose

- **Spiritual**: Grounding practices, prayer, plant medicine (Ayahuasca, Iboga), breathwork

One must **grieve the illusion** of invincibility and reclaim the deeper truths hidden beneath the armor.

Conclusion: Tren as the Shadow Mirror

Trenbolone reveals more about a person than it gives them:

- It shows how far someone is willing to go to feel powerful.

- It exposes wounds hidden beneath the need for control.

- It breaks open the illusion that more muscle equals more love.

Tren is not just a steroid—it is an initiation.

For some, it's a descent into ego death. For others, it's a crucible of reckoning.

But to use Tren spiritually, if at all, is to do so **with sacred intention, deep awareness, and radical honesty.**

My advice, avoid Tren entirely, the risk is not worth the reward.

A Solid Alternative... DHB

DHB (dihydroboldenone, also called 1-testosterone cypionate) is often compared to **trenbolone** because they share certain anabolic traits — but DHB can be a viable alternative when you want **strength and physique enhancement** without some of tren's harsher side effects.

Similarities to Trenbolone

- **High Anabolic:Androgenic Ratio** – Both deliver strong muscle-building effects without excessive estrogen conversion.

- **Lean, Dry Gains** – DHB, like tren, tends to produce hard, vascular muscle without the water retention common to aromatizing compounds.

- **Strength Increase** – Both enhance neural efficiency and power output.

✅ Why DHB Can Be a Better Alternative

1. **Milder Neurological Side Effects**

- Trenbolone is notorious for anxiety, irritability, insomnia, and "tren cough."

- DHB is far less likely to cause extreme mood swings or severe sleep disruption.

2. **Less Impact on Cardio Endurance**

- Tren can significantly impair cardiovascular capacity by raising hematocrit and affecting oxygen transport.

- DHB still affects blood thickness over time but is generally less crippling to cardio output.

3. **Cleaner Appetite Profile**

- Tren often suppresses appetite; DHB is more neutral, allowing better adherence to nutrition plans.

4. **Minimal Progestogenic Activity**

- Tren interacts with progesterone receptors, which can contribute to gyno risk in certain users; DHB's impact here is negligible.

5. **Aesthetic Appeal**

- Produces a similar "grainy," competition-ready look without as much systemic stress.

⚠ Considerations & Downsides

- **Injection Volume & PIP** – DHB is often painful to inject and usually brewed at lower concentrations, requiring larger injection volumes.

- **Erythrocytosis Risk** – Can still raise hematocrit, requiring regular blood monitoring.

- **Liver & Kidney Load** – As with any potent anabolic, organ health must be monitored.

- **Moderate Androgenic Effects** – Still capable of causing hair loss or acne in genetically prone users.

🔄 Ideal Use Case

- **Cutting or Recomp Cycles** where the goal is:

- Lean, dense muscle

- Minimal bloat

- High strength retention in a calorie deficit

- **Bridging Between Heavier Compounds** for athletes who want tren-like hardness without being "fried" by harsh CNS side effects.

🧘 Health-Conscious Strategy

- Cycle length: **8–12 weeks**

- Bloodwork every 6–8 weeks

- Stack with joint-friendly, recovery-supportive peptides (BPC-157, TB-500) and mitochondrial support (CoQ10, MOTS-C, NAD+)

- Use sauna, cardiovascular training, and hydration protocols to support hematocrit and vascular health.

The Shadows Within the Iron Temple

I've witnessed—and lived through—some of the deepest shadows that haunt the world of bodybuilding. It's a realm that demands everything: your time, your focus, your body, your very identity. And if you're not rooted in something deeper than your reflection, it will take more than it gives.

To thrive in this space requires a mind forged from fire—but also a heart protected from corrosion. Because beneath the discipline and the admiration lies a much darker terrain. This is a subculture where **narcissism is currency**, where **overcompensated masculinity becomes armor**, and where the hunger for validation often eclipses the hunger for true well-being.

It's a vortex—seductive and relentless—where loneliness wears many disguises: the grind, the hustle, the pursuit of a perfect physique. Where unresolved pain expresses itself through obsessive routines, sexual escapism, emotional isolation, and the endless need to be *seen*. More often than not, the very tools used to sculpt the body—performance-enhancing drugs, chronic stimulation, the constant pressure to produce and perform—begin to erode the soul.

I've seen it end in **illness, madness, addiction, even death**. I've seen dreams become delusions. And I've felt it myself—the cost of chasing the illusion, the regret of harming others on the way, the numbness that creeps in when you silence your own Spirit for long enough.

What often gets overlooked in this world is just how **energetically violent** it can be to stay in a state of constant "more"—more food, more weight, more testosterone, more approval. This unrelenting Yang energy, when unbalanced by introspection, compassion, or surrender, leads to burnout at best, and spiritual collapse at worst.

I was fortunate—**plant medicine found me** before I lost myself completely. Ayahuasca, Kambo, Bufo, Iboga—they cracked open the shell I had built around my heart and showed me what true strength looks like: the strength to *feel*, to *forgive*, to *let go.* But I didn't come to that healing without hurting people along the way—and without hurting myself.

The industry is beginning to shift. I see more lifters, influencers, and competitors slowly merging the **philosophy of bodybuilding** with the **principles of longevity and inner wellness**. Biohacking, mindfulness, recovery, breath-work—they're being woven into the conversation. But the loudest voices are still the ones glamorizing extremes: the "Tren transformations," the sex-fueled persona-building, the algorithm-chasing workouts filmed for likes instead of self-respect.

And then there's the brutal truth no one wants to say aloud: **genetics determine more than effort ever will.** You can work harder than anyone you know and still fall short. For most, the Pro Card remains just out of reach, and the cost of getting close is often a trail of broken relationships, compromised organs, and disillusionment. I've met thousands of competitors, and maybe 1–2% of the professionals I've known are able to create something truly *healthy* in that world. Most sacrifice too much of themselves along the way.

We glorify ambition, drive, and commitment—but without discernment and spiritual grounding, those virtues become vices. This new generation, enamored with quick results and online attention, is walking a razor's edge. They're burning bright, but burning out faster—crippled by anxiety, haunted by depression, numbed by drugs, and in too many tragic cases, **considering whether life is worth continuing**.

The irony is heartbreaking: these physiques we worship as models of strength are often masks hiding deep pain. And in that disconnect between appearance and reality, we lose something sacred.

This book is a prayer to restore it. To bring back truth, presence, and purpose. To remind us that the body is not a battleground—it's a temple. And what we do with it, what we put into it, and how we carry it... echoes through every layer of who we are becoming.

- Disrupts natural hormonal feedback loops → soul/body misalignment

- Feeds illusion of invincibility

- Loss of sacred timing, grounded humility

Chapter 5: Two Roads – Ego vs. Embodiment

Section A: Egoic/Shadow Path

From Shadow to Sanctuary — Healing the Wounds Beneath the Muscle

Not everyone who enters a gym is chasing gains. Many are running—from memories, from shame, from a sense of unworthiness so ingrained that even muscle can't mask it. While iron has the potential to sculpt strength, confidence, and resilience, it can also become a weapon turned inward, used to punish a body that is seen as flawed, weak, or simply unlovable.

This chapter dives deep into one of the most important and overlooked realities in the world of bodybuilding: that training can be a disguise for deeper wounds. And that without awareness, we may unknowingly harden our bodies while leaving our hearts untouched.

I. The Inner War: When Training Becomes a Battle With Self

1. Self-Hate as Fuel For many, the first rep is not born of inspiration—but desperation. The drive begins with a whisper: "I'm not enough." This internal narrative may be buried beneath grit, discipline, and aesthetics, but it pulses through every lift. Instead of training from a place of self-respect, the athlete trains to become someone else—someone more lovable, more powerful, more accepted.

2. Body Shame and Dissociation In this state, the body is no longer home—it becomes an enemy. A project. A problem to solve. Mirrors don't reflect growth; they reflect inadequacy. Training becomes compulsive, not conscious. Rest is weakness. Pain is dismissed. The connection between mind and body is severed.

3. Trauma as the Hidden Driver Many athletes don't realize that unresolved childhood trauma or emotional wounds are fueling their desire for control. The gym offers a false sense of predictability. Reps and macros offer clarity in a world that felt unsafe or chaotic. This energy may produce discipline—but it's brittle. Eventually, it breaks.

II. The Visible Signs: What Shadow Training Looks Like

To the outside world, it's just "hardcore training." But to those with eyes to see, the symptoms are clear:

- **Ignoring injury or illness:** pushing through pain to meet an emotional quota

- **Disordered eating patterns:** cycling between starvation, bingeing, and obsession

- **Overuse of fat burners, PEDs, and stimulants:** often to numb emotional exhaustion

- **Mirror addiction and body-checking:** never satisfied, always chasing an elusive ideal

- **Emotional volatility:** anger, depression, or identity collapse when progress stalls

This is not discipline. It's dysregulation in disguise.

III. The Energetic and Somatic Toll

Training from a wounded place does not just harm muscles—it harms the nervous system and soul:

- **Sympathetic dominance:** the body remains stuck in fight/flight

- **Adrenal fatigue:** the result of long-term cortisol and stimulant use

- **Muscle armor:** emotional tension stored in the fascia and joints

- **Blocked energy centers:** especially the heart and solar plexus

- **Fragmented self-identity:** "I am only worthy when I'm progressing"

These consequences manifest in anxiety, depression, gut issues, and even autoimmune symptoms—yet they are rarely connected back to the root: a fractured relationship with the self.

IV. Awakening: From Self-Punishment to Self-Compassion

Healing does not require quitting training. It requires changing our orientation to it. When we begin to see the gym as a place to **meet ourselves**, not to **escape ourselves**, everything changes.

From This...	To This...
I train to fix myself	I train to know myself
I punish my body	I partner with my body
I hate my reflection	I honor my evolution
I fear rest	I integrate stillness and healing

V. Tools and Practices for Healing the Inner Athlete

1. Nervous System Recalibration

- Breathwork (e.g., Coherent breathing, Box breathing)

- Cold exposure with intention, not addiction

- Gentle movement practices (yoga, qigong)

2. Somatic and Inner Child Work

- Releasing emotion through body-based therapy

- Identifying the origin of "not enoughness"

- Re-parenting the self with compassion and boundaries

3. Shadow Work

- Journaling prompts to explore envy, fear, and ego

- Meditations to reconnect with body and sensation

4. Plant Medicine (with discernment and ceremony)

- *Ayahuasca*: deep insight into emotional and spiritual wounds

- *Kambo*: cleansing toxic physical and energetic burdens

- *Iboga*: restructuring trauma patterns at their core

- *Bufo*: ego death and rebirth into body-acceptance

VI. Integration: The Sacred Path of Spiritual Bodybuilding

When we reclaim training as a form of **integration**, we fuse strength with softness, discipline with discernment, masculinity with intuition. We no longer chase perfection. We cultivate presence.

True hypertrophy happens not just in the muscle—but in the heart.

To transmute pain into power. To convert shame into sovereignty. To let the body become not a billboard for validation—but a vessel for spirit.

That is the path of the spiritual bodybuilder. And that path begins not with more reps—but with a single question:

Am I training to escape myself—or to meet myself more deeply?

- Obsession with numbers, mirrors, external validation

- Disconnection from feeling, intuition, and Spirit

- Feeds the illusion of control and perfectionism

Section B: Embodied/Mindful Path

Training as a meditative ritual, devotional act:

- Awareness of breath, sensation, intention

- Body as teacher and companion, not enemy

- How this approach **opens the heart** and grounds the psyche

- **Key Teaching**: "The way you lift is the way you live."

Chapter 6: The Shadow of the Iron Path – What Unhealthy Bodybuilding Looks Like

An **unhealthy bodybuilding lifestyle** emerges when the **pursuit of muscle size, leanness, or performance** overrides balance in physiology, psychology, and spirit.

It's not just "lifting too much" — it's the **systematic overdriving of the body's machinery** combined with **neglect of recovery, emotional needs, and internal health signals**.

💧 PHYSICAL CHARACTERISTICS

1. PED Overuse Without Recovery

- Chronic **anabolic steroid** cycles with minimal off-time, stacking multiple compounds.

- **Insulin, GH, IGF-1** abuse leading to organ enlargement, insulin resistance, and possible cancer risk.

- Using **stimulants and fat burners** year-round, blunting adrenal function.

2. Overtraining & Under-Recovery

- High-volume training with insufficient sleep or deload weeks.

- Ignoring signs of injury or chronic inflammation (joints, tendons, fascia).

- Muscle growth prioritized over **lymphatic & glymphatic system health**, leading to toxic buildup.

3. Narrow Nutritional Approach

- Chronic **high-protein, low-micronutrient diets**.

- Reliance on **low-quality supplements** with synthetic fillers.

- Ignoring digestive recovery — leading to gut inflammation, nutrient malabsorption.

4. Neglected Internal Health

- Suppressed natural testosterone, thyroid, or adrenal function.

- Thickened blood (high hematocrit) from PED use → cardiovascular risk.

- Overstressed liver & kidneys from drug, supplement, and protein load.

🧠 MENTAL & EMOTIONAL CHARACTERISTICS

1. Body Dysmorphia & Identity Fusion

- Self-worth tied entirely to physique metrics.

- "Never big enough" or "never lean enough" mindset, no matter progress.

- Anxiety or depression during injury or forced rest periods.

2. Addiction to Extremes

- **Training, diet, and enhancement become compulsive behaviors**.

- Constant need for "the next cycle," "the next peptide," "the next show."

- Fear of losing muscle → reluctance to take rest days or scale back intensity.

3. Emotional Suppression

- Using training and PED-induced dopamine as a way to avoid unresolved trauma.

- Inability to sit with stillness or engage in self-reflection without discomfort.

⟳ BIOCHEMICAL CONSEQUENCES

- **HPA Axis dysfunction** → adrenal burnout.

- **Altered Bohr effect** from chronic stimulant/PED use → impaired oxygen utilization.

- Chronic inflammation disrupting **lymphatic and glymphatic clearance**.

- Hormonal instability causing mood swings, poor sleep, and immune suppression.

- Increased oxidative stress → accelerated cellular aging despite youthful appearance.

⤳ SPIRITUAL IMPLICATIONS

1. Disconnection from Body Wisdom

- Ignoring pain, fatigue, and intuition because the *ego-driven physique goal* is louder.

- Treating the body like a **machine to be forced** rather than a **temple to be cared for**.

2. Ego Over Soul

- Pursuing external validation (stage wins, social media likes) instead of inner fulfillment.

- Muscle mass becomes a **shield** — a way to armor oneself emotionally and spiritually.

3. Suppression of Emotional Detox

- Lymphatic stagnation (from inflammation, PED toxicity) mirrors **emotional stagnation** — old grief, anger, and shame never processed.

- Spiritual growth stalls because **stillness, humility, and receptivity** are replaced by constant output and overexertion.

LONG-TERM TRAJECTORY

- Initially: rapid muscle gain, increased confidence, high energy.

- Mid-term: joint wear, gut dysfunction, reduced natural hormone production, emotional instability.

- Long-term: cardiovascular disease, organ damage, cognitive decline, disconnection from authentic self, and possible spiritual crisis.

IN SHORT

An unhealthy bodybuilding lifestyle is **an imbalanced alchemy**:

- **Physically**: The exterior looks powerful while the interior systems quietly degrade.

- **Mentally**: Discipline morphs into compulsion.

- **Biochemically**: The body is in chronic survival mode.

- **Spiritually**: The soul's voice is drowned out by the ego's demand for "more."

Chapter 7: The Crisis of Early Enhancement (Ages 15–25)

The Weight of Rushing the Journey — The Dangers of Early PED Use (Ages 15–25)

Introduction: A Fork in the Road

The first time a young person contemplates taking a performance-enhancing drug, they stand at a spiritual and biological fork in the road—whether they know it or not. It may seem like a small decision, wrapped in excitement and ambition, but what lies beneath is far more significant: a choice between **natural evolution or artificial acceleration**, between integration or fragmentation.

For those between the ages of **15 and 25**, this decision carries uniquely potent risks. At a time when the brain, hormones, and spiritual identity are still solidifying, introducing synthetic hormones can unravel the very fabric of growth—physically, emotionally, and spiritually.

This chapter explores what happens when we interrupt nature's process too early—and what's truly at stake when we do.

1. The Biology of Becoming: A Body Still in Formation

Between puberty and the mid-twenties, the human endocrine system is engaged in a delicate dance of development.

- The **hypothalamic-pituitary-gonadal (HPG) axis** is calibrating long-term testosterone and fertility rhythms.

- The **epiphyseal growth plates** in bones are still open.

- Brain regions tied to **impulse control, identity, and future planning** are maturing.

- Emotional regulation pathways are still under construction.

Injecting synthetic testosterone or growth hormones during this window doesn't just add fuel to the fire—it can burn the entire house down.

Key Risks:

- **Stunted growth** due to premature closure of growth plates.

- **Infertility** and long-term hypogonadism from shutdown of natural testosterone.

- **Permanent acne, hair loss**, and voice changes (even in young women experimenting with PEDs).

- **Cardiac risks** due to early hypertrophy and elevated LDL cholesterol.

- **Liver strain and toxicity**, especially from oral steroids.

- **Neurochemical disruption**, increasing the likelihood of depression, aggression, and impulsivity.

2. The Psychology of Power: When Identity Forms Around Muscle

At 17, 19, or 22, the body is still becoming—but so is the **self**.

Introducing PEDs during this fragile time can imprint the belief that **who I am is not enough**, that without these substances, I cannot win, cannot attract, cannot be seen.

This is a deep psychological wound—a wound of **conditional worth**.

What often follows:

- **Addiction to validation**: The mirror becomes a weapon. Without a pump, without fullness, the individual spirals into insecurity.

- **Muscle dysmorphia**: A distorted body image where no level of mass is ever sufficient.

- **Emotional volatility**: PEDs heighten aggression, decrease emotional stability, and amplify shame in post-cycle crashes.

- **Social isolation**: As the body becomes a mask, intimacy and vulnerability fade. People love the image, not the soul inside it.

3. The Spiritual Crisis: When Artificial Fire Burns the Temple

The spiritual implications of early PED use are often the least discussed—but perhaps the most important.

When a young bodybuilder floods their system with synthetic hormones, they override the body's sacred rhythm. In doing so, they often lose **connection to their inner wisdom**.

Spiritual Consequences:

- **Loss of inner listening**: PEDs numb subtle cues. Pain is ignored. Rest is dismissed. The inner voice becomes irrelevant.

- **Ego dominance**: The body becomes an idol. Performance and aesthetics replace purpose and presence.

- **Energetic imbalance**: Chronic high-androgen states inflame the solar plexus (ego center), overstimulate the adrenals, and fragment the heart-space.

- **Blocked awakening**: Spiritual growth requires softness, vulnerability, and surrender. PEDs harden the body—and often the soul.

For some, this journey ends in tragedy: **overdose, suicide, irreversible health decline**, or total disillusionment. For others, the symptoms are quieter but no less painful: fatigue, shame, emotional repression, and a gnawing sense that the soul was left behind in pursuit of a fleeting ideal.

4. The Cultural Mirage: Tren, TikTok, and the New Gladiator

Today's digital culture adds another layer of danger.

Social media platforms like TikTok, Instagram, and YouTube flood young minds with:

- **Fake natty influencers**

- **"Before-and-after" transformations**

- **Glamorization of extreme drug cycles (e.g., Trenbolone)**

In this culture, PEDs are no longer taboo—they're celebrated, memed, and monetized. The sacredness of the body is reduced to algorithm-driven content, while the soul drowns in dopamine hits from likes and comments.

But behind the filtered perfection lies a truth few talk about:

- The **panic attacks**

- The **crashes in self-worth**

- The **broken endocrine systems**

- The **lost spiritual anchors**

This mirage has cost many young men and women their joy, their health, and sometimes their lives.

5. The Way of Wisdom: Delayed Gratification and Sacred Discipline

To say **no** to PEDs in your teens and twenties is not weakness—it's wisdom. It is choosing to walk the **long path**, the one that forges character alongside muscle, clarity alongside strength.

This is the path of the **Spiritual Bodybuilder**.

It means:

- Learning the body's natural rhythms.

- Cultivating patience, consistency, and self-love.

- Building strength from the inside out.

- Seeking spiritual alignment, not just symmetry.

When you wait, when you grow naturally, when you **earn** your body through presence, breath, and ritual—you gain more than mass. You gain mastery.

6. A Better Alternative: Integration Over Domination

What to focus on instead of early PED use:

- **Nutrition**: Balance, timing, gut health, and spiritual nourishment.

- **Training**: Periodization, progressive overload, mind-muscle connection.

- **Recovery**: Sleep, breathwork, emotional regulation, nervous system health.

- **Mindset**: Therapy, journaling, emotional intelligence work.

- **Spiritual Practice**: Meditation, plant medicine (when mature and ready), inner child work, connection to nature.

Conclusion: Your Temple, Your Timing

Your body is not a race car to be redlined at 17. It is a **temple**, a living altar, and your sacred home. Every hormone, every muscle fiber, every breath—it all forms a dialogue between flesh and spirit.

To rush this process is to rob yourself of the **most profound journey** a young person can undertake: the slow, patient unfolding of potential into purpose, strength into stewardship, and power into peace.

When you walk the path of restraint, self-respect, and spiritual embodiment, you don't just build a physique—you build a legacy of wholeness.

- Dangers of using steroids too early:
    - Hormonal axis not fully developed
    - Brain (especially prefrontal cortex) still maturing
- Spiritual consequences:
    - Incomplete soul integration with the body
    - Ego inflates before wisdom anchors
    - Delayed maturity, loss of inner authority, emotional disconnection

Chapter 8: The Sacred Science of Enhancement — Exploring PEDs with Wisdom and Maturity

There comes a moment for many who walk the path of spiritual bodybuilding when they begin to contemplate performance enhancement not from a place of lack or insecurity, but from curiosity, wisdom, and integration.

The body is more resilient, the mind more stable, and the spirit more anchored. When approached consciously, Performance Enhancing Drugs (PEDs) can become tools for deepened embodiment and evolution—*not shortcuts*, but sacred tools applied with reverence and awareness.

This chapter offers a detailed roadmap for those over 25 seeking to explore PEDs safely. We will break it down into two age ranges—**25 to 40** and **41 to 60**—and explore specific biomarkers, emotional checkpoints, and spiritual prerequisites for each.

Section I: Age 25 to 40 — Grounded Expansion

By the mid-twenties, the endocrine system has matured, the brain has solidified its executive function, and the emotional body is (ideally) more regulated. This age range offers fertile ground for responsible, bio-informed enhancement.

Why This Age Range Matters

- Natural testosterone has reached its peak and may slowly begin to decline.

- Neurological and cardiovascular systems are still highly adaptable.

- Recovery capacity is strong if well-nourished.

Before You Begin: Non-Negotiable Foundations

- **Stable diet and gut health**

- **Consistent sleep cycles (7-9 hrs)**

- **Proven training history (minimum 5+ years of lifting)**

- **Emotional intelligence and support system in place**

- **Zero need for external validation**

Spiritual Readiness Questions

- Can you walk away from the mirror without judgment?

- Are you willing to track your health more than your appearance?

- Can you handle strength without ego?

Section II: Age 41 to 60 — Longevity, Vitality & Sacred Stewardship

This is the phase of **alchemical maturity**. The desire to optimize becomes less about dominance and more about **quality of life, recovery, cognition, and resilience**.

Why This Age Range is Critical

- Natural testosterone declines ~1% per year after 30

- Recovery slows

- Muscle protein synthesis decreases

- Cognitive clarity and libido may wane

Essential Lab Markers Before Considering PEDs

- **Testosterone Panel** (Total, Free, SHBG, Bioavailable)

- **DHEA-S**: Master adrenal hormone

- **Cortisol (AM/PM)**: Check stress response

- **IGF-1**: Growth hormone surrogate

- **Homocysteine**: Heart health + methylation

- **Vitamin D3, B12, and Ferritin**: Nutrient baselines

- **PSA** (men): Prostate health

- **Thyroid Panel** (TSH, FT3, FT4, RT3)

Optimal Enhancements (with monitoring)

- **TRT**: 100-250mg/week

- **HCG**: To maintain fertility and natural function

- **HGH or Peptides (Epithalon, CJC-1295/Ipamorelin)**

- **NAD+ Therapy**: Mitochondrial restoration

- **GLP-1, Metformin or Berberine**: Insulin sensitivity support

- Customized **Peptide protocol** based on current state of health

Mind/Body Integration Practices

- **Breathwork and cold exposure** to support neuroendocrine tone

- **Qi Gong or Kundalini Yoga** to awaken life force

- **Plant medicine integration (Ayahuasca, Iboga, Kambo)** for detox and psycho-spiritual realignment

- **Emotional somatic therapy** to unravel performance-based identity

Spiritual Disciplines for This Phase

- Redefining masculinity/femininity through *service*, not dominance

- Offering wisdom to the younger generation

- Building strength as a temple, not a trophy

Red Flags — When Not to Start PEDs

- Emotional volatility or unresolved trauma

- Inconsistent lifestyle habits (sleep, diet, training)

- No established healthcare provider or coach

- Motivated primarily by social media image

- History of addiction, compulsive behavior, or depression (without support)

Closing: The Alchemy of Conscious Enhancement

PEDs are not evil. They are **tools**. And like all tools, they magnify the hand that wields them.

Used unconsciously, they can destroy a life. Used consciously, they can enhance one.

The question is not *"Should I take PEDs?"* but rather:

- **"Am I ready to be a steward of power?"**

- **"Am I in right relationship with my body, my ego, and my spirit?"**

When the answer is yes—and only then—the path opens.

And it becomes not just a path of enhancement, but of **elevation.**

- Centered in **self-love, ritual, and inner harmony**

- PED use (if any) done with **discernment, mentorship, lab data, and reverence**

- Connection to **natural cycles**: sleep, sun, seasons, rest

- Integration of practices like:

- Meditation

- Cold exposure

- Somatic release

- Breathwork

- Plant medicine (optional spiritual support)

🧬 Aging, Bodybuilding, and Performance: 25–40 vs. 41–60

⚡ Hormonal Environment

Age 25–40

- Testosterone, GH, and IGF-1 are near peak (unless suppressed by lifestyle or PED abuse).

- Recovery is faster; anabolic signaling is more efficient.

- PEDs and peptides often yield **rapid gains** with relatively less collateral damage.

Age 41–60

- Gradual decline in testosterone and GH/IGF-1.

- Cortisol sensitivity increases; stress recovery is slower.

- Estrogen, prolactin, and SHBG shifts complicate balance.

- PEDs can still be used, but need to be **lower dose, more precise, and health-focused**, often blending with TRT and peptide therapies.

🏋 Training Considerations

Age 25–40

- Can tolerate higher volume and intensity (more heavy lifting, HIIT, failure training).

- Focus: hypertrophy, strength, pushing limits.

- Recovery capacity = high; connective tissues are more forgiving.

Age 41–60

- Greater focus on **joint preservation, mobility, and recovery**.

- Prioritize **quality over quantity** — tempo, time under tension, perfect form.

- Deloads and active recovery become essential.

- Focus shifts toward maintaining **muscle density, functional strength, and metabolic health**.

✎ Performance Enhancement & Biohacking

Age 25–40

- Steroids, SARMs, and GH can be used more aggressively — though risks accumulate long-term.

- Focus on **muscle building and performance maximization**.

- Biohacks: intermittent fasting, sauna/ice, basic peptides (BPC-157, TB-500).

Age 41–60

- Precision > power.

- TRT often replaces high-dose steroid cycles.

- Peptides play a larger role: **CJC-1295/Ipamorelin, BPC-157, Thymosins, MOTS-C, Epithalon** for repair and longevity.

- Mitochondrial support becomes critical: **CoQ10, SS-31, NAD+ boosters**.

- Biohacks shift toward **hormetic stress with recovery**: breathwork, fasting-mimicking diets, circadian alignment, HRV monitoring.

⚕ Health Risks & Markers

Age 25–40

- Main risks: liver strain (oral steroids), blood pressure, acne, sleep disturbance.

- Bloodwork focus: liver enzymes, hematocrit, lipids, testosterone/estradiol.

Age 41–60

- Risks expand: cardiovascular disease, insulin resistance, kidney strain, cognitive decline.

- Bloodwork focus:

- **Liver/kidney panels**

- **Cardiac markers** (lipids, ApoB, hs-CRP, calcium score)

- **Thyroid panel** (TSH, Free T3, rT3, antibodies)

- **Hormone panel** (T, SHBG, DHEA-S, cortisol, estradiol)

- **IGF-1** (keep in high-normal but not supra-physiologic range).

🧘 Mindset & Emotional Shifts

Age 25-40

- Driven by growth, pushing limits, external validation (stage wins, PRs, aesthetics).

- More resilient psychologically to overtraining and extremes.

Age 41-60

- Shift toward **sustainability, balance, longevity**.

- Training becomes about vitality, mobility, and *enjoying the body as a temple*, not punishing it.

- Emotional mastery and spiritual connection play a much larger role — bodybuilding as meditation, discipline, and health.

🚫 What to Avoid

25-40

- Chronic stimulant use.

- Ignoring recovery or bloodwork.

- "Blast and cruise" mentality with no endgame.

41-60

- High-dose steroid cycles (major cardiovascular risk).

- Chronic caloric restriction (leads to muscle/fatigue issues).

- Neglecting cardiovascular and brain health.

- Overtraining heavy compound lifts without balancing mobility and recovery.

✅ What to Focus On

<u>25–40</u>

- Building mass and strength as a "bank" for later years.

- Experimentation with biohacks and PEDs — but keep health safeguards in place.

- Optimizing recovery habits early (sleep, nutrition, stress management).

<u>41–60</u>

- Preserving lean mass, bone density, and metabolic health.

- Supporting hormone balance through TRT/peptides/nutrition.

- Mitochondrial health, inflammation control, cardiovascular conditioning.

- Shifting from ego-driven bodybuilding to **longevity-driven bodybuilding**.

✨ Summary

- **25–40**: Build, experiment, push — but set the foundation for health.

- **41–60**: Refine, protect, balance — longevity and vitality become the new PRs.

Bodybuilding evolves from **maximum growth** to **sustainable strength**, from **ego-driven performance** to **spirit-driven vitality**.

🏋️ Training Principles After 60

<u>Prioritize Strength & Function</u>

- Continue lifting heavy, but focus on **moderate loads with excellent form** rather than chasing PRs.

- Emphasize **compound lifts** (squats, deadlifts, presses, pulls) at submaximal intensity to maintain muscle, bone density, and CNS health.

Mobility & Stability First

- Add regular mobility drills, yoga, and prehab work to protect joints.

- Core stability and balance training reduce fall risk and preserve athleticism.

Volume & Recovery

- Lower training volume compared to earlier years, but stay **consistent** (3–4 strength sessions per week).

- Incorporate active recovery: walking, swimming, light cycling, sauna, stretching.

Hormone & Biochemical Health

Testosterone Support

- Many men over 60 benefit from carefully monitored **TRT**, keeping testosterone in the high-normal range for age.

- Avoid supra-physiological dosing — the goal is *vitality and function*, not aggressive hypertrophy.

Peptide Therapies

- **CJC-1295/Ipamorelin**: restore GH pulsatility for recovery and fat metabolism.

- **BPC-157, TB-500**: support tissue healing and injury prevention.

- **MOTS-C, SS-31, Epithalon**: enhance mitochondrial function and longevity.

Thyroid Monitoring

- Ensure Free T3, Free T4, and TSH are optimal, as thyroid decline is common with age.

IGF-1 Optimization

- Aim for mid–high normal (120–180 ng/mL depending on age), avoiding high-risk supraphysiologic ranges.

🍽 Nutrition & Gut Health

Protein Intake

- Maintain **1.2–1.6 g protein/kg bodyweight** daily to preserve lean mass.

- Use easy-to-digest proteins (collagen, whey isolate, eggs, fish) to reduce gut strain.

Micronutrient Density

- Prioritize magnesium, zinc, vitamin D, selenium, B vitamins.

- Use whole-food based supplementation to support hormones, recovery, and mitochondria.

Gut & Liver Support

- Probiotics, fiber, and cruciferous vegetables for digestion and detox.

- TUDCA or NAC for liver health if on long-term medications or TRT.

🖤 Cardiovascular & Cognitive Health

Cardio Training

- 2–3 sessions/week of **zone 2 cardio** (walking, cycling, rowing) for heart and metabolic health.

- Add short HIIT sessions occasionally for mitochondrial resilience.

Bloodwork Monitoring

- Kidney and liver panels, lipid profile, hs-CRP, fasting insulin, HbA1c.

- Testosterone, estradiol, SHBG, thyroid panel, IGF-1.

- Check cardiovascular markers (ApoB, Lipoprotein(a), CAC scan if risk factors present).

Cognitive Preservation

- Prioritize sleep, meditation, red light therapy, and neuroprotective peptides (Semax, Selank, Dihexa).

Mindset & Spiritual Integration

- Shift the goal from **maximal physique** to **sustainable strength and longevity**.

- Use training as meditation: each rep as presence, each workout as ritual.

- Value **energy, clarity, and resilience** over sheer size.

- Reframe bodybuilding as a vehicle for vitality and connection, not competition.

What to Avoid After 60

- High-dose steroid cycles (increases risk of CVD, kidney disease, and cancer).

- Chronic stimulant use (fat burners, clenbuterol, excessive caffeine).

- Overtraining heavy compound lifts without joint care.

- Extreme diets that deplete recovery and hormones.

☑ What to Focus On

- Resistance training for **lean mass and bone density**.

- Longevity-focused biohacks: sauna, breathwork, sleep optimization, fasting-mimicking diets.

- Precision medicine: low-dose TRT/peptides, tailored supplements, and regular labs.

- Balance: bodybuilding as meditation and spiritual practice, not ego-driven performance.

✦ **In summary**: After 60, the best approach is to **train smart, recover deeply, support hormones responsibly, and shift from "growth at all costs" to "strength with longevity."** The body becomes both the temple and the teacher — guiding you toward health, resilience, and inner mastery.

41-60 VS. 60+

⚖ Training

41–60

- Still capable of moderate-high intensity, but with more structured deloads.

- Goal = **maintain size, strength, and functionality**, while respecting slower recovery.

- Heavy compound lifts are still central, but balanced with mobility work.

60+

- Shift from **maximum output** to **safe longevity lifting**.

- Moderate loads with **perfect form** prioritized over intensity.

- Greater emphasis on **joint health, stability, balance, and injury prevention**.

- Consistency matters more than intensity — the body thrives on rhythm and sustainability.

Hormones & Enhancement

41–60

- Many men begin **TRT** as natural testosterone declines.

- Peptides like **CJC-1295/Ipamorelin, BPC-157, Thymosins** support recovery and lean mass.

- Some may still experiment with lower-dose PEDs, but with health monitoring.

60+

- The goal is no longer maximizing anabolism but **preserving hormonal balance**.

- **Low-dose TRT** is often continued, carefully monitored to avoid cardiovascular stress.

- Peptides shift toward **regeneration and mitochondrial support**: MOTS-C, SS-31, Epithalon.

- **High-dose PEDs are contraindicated** due to cardiovascular and cancer risks.

Nutrition

41–60

- Macronutrient cycling (higher protein, strategic carbs/fats) supports strength and recovery.

- Focus on keeping visceral fat low to maintain insulin sensitivity.

<u>60+</u>

- Protein remains essential (1.2–1.6 g/kg), but **digestibility and gut health** become priority.

- Micronutrient density, liver support, and anti-inflammatory foods dominate.

- Caloric balance favors **sustainability** — enough to preserve mass, not excess to strain organs.

🩶 Cardiovascular & Cognitive Health

<u>41–60</u>

- Cardio is used as a supplement to lifting — typically 2–3 times per week.

- Bloodwork checks include lipids, glucose control, liver/kidney, thyroid.

<u>60+</u>

- Cardio becomes **equally important to resistance training**: zone 2 cardio for heart and brain health, plus balance/coordination drills.

- More advanced screenings recommended: **CAC scans, ApoB, Lipoprotein(a), hs-CRP**.

- Cognitive support (sleep, red light therapy, neuroprotective peptides like Semax/Selank).

🧘 Mindset & Spiritual Focus

<u>41–60</u>

- Shift from ego-driven training toward **longevity and balance**.

- Training reframed as a sustainable lifestyle.

<u>60+</u>

- Bodybuilding becomes **medicine and meditation**.

- The gym = a temple for maintaining life-force, not for chasing size.

- Spiritual practice integrates with lifting: resilience, humility, gratitude for movement itself.

🚫 What to Avoid

- **41–60**: avoid high-dose cycles, overtraining, chronic stimulants.

- **60+**: avoid aggressive PEDs altogether, extreme diets, or punishing volume/intensity. Joint-destroying lifts and ego-based training should be left behind.

✅ The Core Difference

- **41–60**: "Preserve what you built, refine it, extend your performance window."

- **60+**: "Protect your temple, sustain your strength, and prioritize vitality, clarity, and longevity over size or power."

✴ In short: 41–60 is about **transitioning from growth to preservation**, while 60+ is about **training for resilience, vitality, and the joy of movement itself.**

🏋 Lifespan Bodybuilding Roadmap

Phase	Age 25–40	Age 41–60	Age 60+
Training	Build foundation: hypertrophy, strength, high intensity; fast recovery allows experimentation.	Preserve & refine: moderate-heavy loads, more mobility, structured deloads, avoid ego lifting.	Longevity lifting: moderate loads, impeccable form, joint & balance focus, rhythm over intensity.

Hormones & Enhancement	Natural T/GH high; some PED use tolerated but risks accumulate; peptides optional.	TRT often begins; peptides (CJC-1295, BPC-157, MOTS-C) support repair & balance; avoid aggressive PED cycles.	Low-dose TRT as foundation; regenerative peptides (MOTS-C, SS-31, Epithalon); avoid anabolic PEDs.
Nutrition	High protein (1.6–2.0 g/kg), carb cycling, surplus/deficit phases for growth or cut.	Maintain lean mass & insulin sensitivity; balanced macros; minimize visceral fat.	Protein 1.2–1.6 g/kg with digestible sources; micronutrient density; anti-inflammatory, gut & liver support.
Recovery	Quick adaptation; recovery often overlooked.	Recovery now equal in importance to training; sauna, ice, breathwork, HRV monitoring.	Recovery is priority; daily mobility, sleep, light cardio, joint care rituals.
Cardiovascular Health	Cardio secondary; HIIT and performance-driven conditioning.	Zone 2 cardio 2–3x/week; HRV and lipid monitoring.	Cardio = longevity tool: zone 2, balance, coordination; CAC scans, ApoB checks.
Cognition & Hormones	Sharp mental resilience; little focus on neuroprotection.	Begin cognitive support: stress management, sleep optimization, red light, Semax/Selank.	Neuroprotection = priority: sleep hygiene, meditation, neuropeptides, social connection.
Mindset & Spirit	Ego-driven goals: size, PRs, competition.	Balance: train for longevity, vitality, functional performance.	Integration: bodybuilding as meditation, resilience, gratitude; focus on vitality, clarity, presence.
What to Avoid	Chronic PED cycles, stimulant abuse, ignoring recovery.	High-dose steroids, overtraining, chronic inflammation, neglecting bloodwork.	Any aggressive PED cycles, punishing intensity, extreme diets, joint-destructive training.

✦ Core Takeaway

- **25–40** = Build → maximize growth, experiment, create foundation.

- **41–60** = Preserve → refine strength, balance hormones, train smart.

- **60+** = Protect → longevity, vitality, clarity, and spiritual integration.

Bodybuilding across the lifespan is less about chasing the heaviest lift or the biggest pump, and more about **evolving goals in harmony with the body's changing rhythms**.

Chapter 9: Gut, Growth, and the Soul – Nutrition as Alchemical Fuel

A. Understanding the Microbiome

To understand the landscape of gut health and what to look for, we must recognize the fundamental philosophy of where science was and where its come to now. The famous debate at the beginning of the Industrial Revolution, Terrain Theory Vs. Germ Theory.

The **difference between terrain theory and germ theory** lies at the heart of one of the most pivotal debates in the history of medicine—a debate that deeply influenced the **rise of modern healthcare**, especially during the **Industrial Revolution**.

This wasn't just a disagreement between two scientific theories. It was a clash of worldviews: one that saw disease as caused by **invading external agents**, and one that believed illness arises from **imbalances within the body and environment**.

Germ Theory: The Invader Model

<u>Pioneers:</u>

- **Louis Pasteur** (France)

- **Robert Koch** (Germany)

Core Belief:

Microorganisms (germs)—like bacteria, viruses, fungi—**cause disease** when they invade a host.

Key Points:

- Disease is **external** in origin.

- Germs are **specific** to diseases (e.g., *Mycobacterium tuberculosis* causes TB).

- Prevention = **sterilization, sanitation, vaccination**.

- Treatment = **drugs that kill or control the microbe** (antibiotics, antivirals, etc.).

This theory became the **foundation of Western medicine**, especially as microscopes advanced and the industrial world needed quick, scalable disease-control methods during epidemics like cholera, typhoid, and tuberculosis.

🦅 Terrain Theory: The Internal Ecosystem Model

Pioneers:

- **Claude Bernard** (France)

- **Antoine Béchamp** (France) – often positioned as Pasteur's philosophical opponent

Core Belief:

Disease results when the body's internal environment (the "terrain") becomes unbalanced or toxic, allowing microbes (which are often already present in the body) to become pathogenic.

Key Points:

- The **body is not sterile**, and microbes are part of the natural ecology.

- Disease = a **result**, not a cause—microbes exploit weakened systems.

- Prevention = **clean nutrition, detoxification, emotional balance, environmental health**.

- Treatment = **strengthening the terrain** rather than attacking the germ.

🏭 The Industrial Revolution Context

During the **19th century**, cities were booming—but with them came:

- Overcrowding

- Poor sanitation

- Pollution

- Malnutrition

- Harsh working conditions

These were ideal conditions for infectious diseases to spread.

Why Germ Theory Triumphed:

- It offered **clear, targeted action**: kill the germ, stop the disease.

- It supported **medical intervention and pharmaceutical development**.

- It was easier to **standardize** and **commercialize**.

- It aligned with the needs of industrial society: **fast, mechanized solutions** to keep the workforce functioning.

Terrain theory, though holistic and preventative, was **slower and more individualized**, and lacked the dramatic "silver bullet" appeal of antibiotics or vaccines.

Pasteur's Later Words (Allegedly):

Near the end of his life, Louis Pasteur is rumored to have said:

"The microbe is nothing. The terrain is everything."

Though unconfirmed, this reflects a softening of his earlier stance and hints at the validity of the terrain-based view.

🌐 Legacy and Modern Revival

Today, many holistic and integrative health systems (functional medicine, naturopathy, Ayurveda, etc.) draw from **terrain theory principles**, focusing on:

- Gut health

- Toxin elimination

- Nutrient sufficiency

- Emotional and energetic balance

Even **Western medicine** is shifting subtly:

- Acknowledging the **microbiome's role** in immunity and disease

- Recognizing how **chronic inflammation, stress, and diet** shape disease outcomes

- Exploring **epigenetics**, where lifestyle shapes gene expression

⚖️ Summary: Germ vs. Terrain

Concept	Germ Theory	Terrain Theory
Cause of Disease	External pathogens	Internal imbalance
Prevention	Sanitize, vaccinate	Detox, nourish, balance

Treatment	Drugs, antibiotics	Support immune system, lifestyle change
Dominant In	Conventional medicine	Holistic and integrative health
Industrial Fit	Mass-scale, rapid action	Personalized, preventative care

Epigenetics: Decoding the microbiome to optimize performance, physically emotionally and spiritually.

Epigenetics is the study of how **external factors**—like environment, lifestyle, diet, stress, and toxins—**influence gene expression** *without changing the underlying DNA sequence*. It shows that genes are not destiny, but rather **dynamic and responsive** to the internal and external environment.

This directly supports **terrain theory**, which emphasizes the **condition of the body's internal environment** (the "terrain") as the key factor in whether disease manifests or healing occurs.

What Is Epigenetics?

Your DNA is like the hardware of a computer. Epigenetics is the **software layer**—it determines which genes are **turned on or off**, and **when**.

Epigenetic changes occur through:

- **DNA methylation** – adding tags that silence or activate genes

- **Histone modification** – altering how tightly DNA is wound, affecting accessibility

- **Non-coding RNAs** – regulating gene activity without altering DNA

These changes are influenced by:

- **Diet** (e.g., folate, polyphenols, glucose levels)

- **Toxins** (heavy metals, endocrine disruptors)

- **Stress** (chronic cortisol alters methylation)

- **Sleep and circadian rhythms**

- **Movement and exercise**

- **Microbiome balance**

- **Trauma and emotional states**

How Epigenetics Supports Terrain Theory

Terrain theory proposes that illness arises when the body's internal environment becomes imbalanced or toxic—conditions under which microbes or dysfunction can thrive.

Epigenetics proves this idea scientifically, by showing that:

- The **biological terrain (e.g., inflammation, nutrient status, oxidative stress)** controls which genes get expressed

- Environmental changes can **activate disease-causing genes** or **silence protective ones**

- You can **influence your health trajectory** by optimizing your inner and outer environment

Examples:
- Chronic stress doesn't change your DNA—but it can **turn on genes linked to anxiety, depression, or inflammation**

- A nutrient-poor diet can silence **tumor suppressor genes**, increasing cancer risk

- Exercise, sleep, and fasting can **upregulate genes** involved in cellular repair and longevity

Epigenetics Is Reversible

Unlike mutations, **epigenetic marks can be modified**. That means:

- Healing is **possible** through terrain-focused practices

- Health isn't just genetic fate—it's a **daily negotiation** between your choices and your genes

This brings the power of health **back to the individual**, aligning perfectly with terrain theory's emphasis on **prevention, nourishment, and balance**.

Final Thought

Epigenetics is the biological mechanism that validates terrain theory.

It shows that your health is not simply written in your genes, but shaped by how you live, what you consume, and how you respond to the world.

Your terrain isn't just soil for your cells—it's a living, responsive **field of possibility**.

Knowing what we know now about how the gut works, we see that it is also Pleomorphic in nature, meaning it changes and shifts according to its environment. Stress, Performance Enhancing Drugs, Overtraining, even massages will shift the tone of the environment. I say all this to emphasize the importance of getting your Microbiome tested. I personally use the VIOME test.

Above all else, if you want to be successful at getting in the best shape of your life, eating the right foods AND making sure they are breaking down and absorbing are equally important factor to consider.

🧬 What Is the Viome Test?

There are several versions of Viome's test, including:

- **Gut Intelligence Test** – Focuses on the gut microbiome only.

- **Health Intelligence Test** – Adds blood analysis for mitochondrial and cellular health.

- **Full Body Intelligence Test** – Includes oral, gut, and cellular health.

Samples are collected at home (via **stool**, **saliva**, and sometimes **blood**) and sent to Viome's lab. There, they use advanced **RNA sequencing (transcriptomics)**—not just DNA—to assess **what your microbes and cells are actually doing right now**.

🧠 What Information Does Viome Provide?

1. Gut Microbiome Activity

- Identifies **which microbes are active**, not just present

- Detects levels of **inflammation, bacterial balance, digestive efficiency**, and **short-chain fatty acid production**

- Flags harmful patterns like **leaky gut, candida overgrowth**, or **histamine intolerance**

2. Mitochondrial and Cellular Health

- Evaluates how well your **mitochondria** (your cells' energy factories) are functioning

- Measures **biological aging** and **cellular stress**

- Can detect **poor detoxification, oxidative stress**, and **inflammation pathways**

3. Oral Microbiome (if included)

- Assesses bacteria in your mouth that can affect **heart health**, **gut health**, and **cognitive function**

🍎 How It Helps You Heal with Personalized Nutrition

Viome doesn't offer generic diets—it creates a **unique food plan tailored to your body's internal signals**. It categorizes foods into:

- **Superfoods** – foods that actively support your current biological needs

- **Enjoy** – foods that are fine in moderation

- **Minimize** – foods to reduce

- **Avoid** – foods that may cause inflammation, fermentation, or stress in your system

Viome may recommend:

- More polyphenols if your oxidative stress is high

- Avoiding turmeric if your sulfur metabolism is impaired

- Avoiding spinach if your oxalate-processing pathways are weak

This **precision nutrition** can help:

- Restore gut balance

- Improve mental clarity and mood

- Reduce chronic inflammation

- Boost energy and mitochondrial performance

- Regulate blood sugar, metabolism, and cravings

Custom Supplement Recommendations

Viome also offers:

- **Precision Supplements** – custom-blended vitamins, minerals, herbs, amino acids, and probiotics based on your test results

- Supplements that are **formulated to support your actual gene expression and microbial function**, not just blanket wellness goals

Healing Body and Mind Through Data

Because the **gut-brain axis** is central to health, Viome's insights can help with:

- **Anxiety and depression** (by improving neurotransmitter precursors and gut health)

- **Focus and cognition** (via mitochondrial and cellular optimization)

- **Sleep regulation** (via nutrient and hormone support)

- **Immune resilience** (by addressing inflammation at the source)

Retesting and Ongoing Adaptation

Your biology is **dynamic**, the microbiome is pleomorphic in nature, meaning it changes in accordance to what its exposed to in its environment, so Viome encourages **retesting every 3–6 months** to:

- See what's improving

- Adjust your diet as your internal environment shifts

- Track reduction in biological age, inflammation, and symptom patterns

🧠 Final Thought

Viome is like giving your body a voice. Instead of guessing which diet or supplement is right, it helps you **listen to your biology's unique language**, revealing what helps you thrive and what quietly drains you.

B. Force-Feeding and the Soul

The Burden of Endless Growth: Breaking the Bulk-At-All-Costs Spell

In modern bodybuilding culture, the "bulk at all costs" mentality has become a near-sacred ritual. A phase defined by force-feeding, rapid size gain, and the obsessive pursuit of numbers—on the scale, in the mirror, and on the plate. For many, it's considered a badge of honor: to push past hunger cues, ignore digestive discomfort, and override the body's natural signals for the sake of "growth."

But beneath this hyper-masculine ethos lies a **spiritual distortion**—a belief that **more is always better** and that **growth must be constant, linear, and aggressive**.

This belief mirrors a deeper collective wound in our society: **the rejection of the feminine principle of rest, integration, and inward reflection**. Just as the Earth moves through seasons—growth, harvest, death, and renewal—the human body and spirit thrive in cycles. But the bulk-at-all-costs approach disrespects this truth, enforcing endless summer, endless sun, endless yang.

"When we force constant growth, we reject nature's wisdom. We become spiritually imbalanced—overfed and undernourished."

Biological Force vs. Intuitive Flow

To bulk often means **suppressing satiety signals**, numbing the body's whispers of discomfort, and seeing digestion not as a sacred alchemical process, but a mechanical funnel for macronutrients.

Meal after meal, the body tries to speak:

- Bloating

- Acid reflux

- Constipation

- Brain fog

- Fatigue

But instead of listening, the athlete doubles down:

"Hit your macros. Eat through the pain. Size is everything."

This is where **intuition begins to erode**. Hunger becomes a number. Satisfaction becomes irrelevant. And the sacred connection to one's own body—the birthplace of inner sovereignty—is severed.

Spiritual Implications: Consumption Without Integration

This relentless mode of overconsumption doesn't only impact the body—it mirrors a **spiritual pattern of consuming life without digesting it**.

We binge food the way we binge experience:

- Chasing stimulus after stimulus

- Avoiding stillness, silence, solitude

- Refusing to metabolize the lessons life offers us

In this way, **force-feeding becomes a metaphor for our disembodied culture**:

- We **grasp** but don't **receive**

- We **acquire** but don't **assimilate**

- We **consume** but don't **contemplate**

"If we don't allow time to digest what we consume—be it food or experience—we stagnate spiritually."

Just as undigested food ferments in the gut, undigested emotion festers in the psyche. We become constipated with unresolved grief, pride, or shame, and no amount of muscle mass can protect us from that inner toxicity.

Reclaiming Balance: The Sacred Pause

True growth is not linear. It's **spiral**. It requires:

- **Expansion and contraction**

- **Consumption and fasting**

- **Effort and surrender**

- **Noise and silence**

Even the best hypertrophy programs are built on cycles: progressive overload, deload, rest. The same must be true for our spiritual lives.

To train, to grow, to feed the body is beautiful. But without cycles of **pause, integration, detoxification, and emotional digestion**, the body becomes inflamed, the mind becomes agitated, and the soul becomes silent.

The sacred pause is where we listen.

The sacred pause is where we heal.

A New Paradigm: Eating with Reverence, Growing with Awareness

Let us shift the narrative from **bulking as domination** to **bulking as nourishment—** from pushing the body to listening to it.

Let us view food not just as fuel, but as **medicine** and **message**—an invitation to connect with the Earth, with ourselves, and with the unseen world.

Let our physical growth not be a rejection of our limitations, but a **celebration of our integration**—where muscle becomes an offering, not an escape.

In this way, bodybuilding becomes not a conquest—but a communion.

C. When Digestion Suffers – Recognizing the Signs

The Burnout of the Inner Flame: Digestive Fire and Spiritual Clarity

In ancient healing traditions—particularly in Ayurveda and Chinese Medicine—the digestive system is viewed not merely as a physical mechanism, but as the **seat of our internal fire**, the **core of vitality**, and a **mirror of spiritual discernment**. When this fire—known as *Agni* or digestive force—is strong, we feel energized, clear, connected. But when it is burned out, both body and spirit suffer.

This concept is more than metaphor. In modern terms, burnout of the digestive system manifests through a range of physiological disruptions—each of which tells a deeper story of spiritual misalignment and emotional exhaustion.

Low Stomach Acid (Hypochlorhydria): The Fire Goes Out

Stomach acid (hydrochloric acid) is a critical initiator of digestion. Without it, proteins go undigested, minerals aren't absorbed, and pathogens remain unchecked. Despite popular misconception, many digestive symptoms stem not from *too much* acid, but from too little.

Symptoms:

- Bloating and heaviness after meals

- Belching or bad breath

- Undigested food in stool

- Low energy or brain fog after eating

Spiritual Parallel:

When the fire within weakens, so does our **clarity**. We lose the ability to *break down experience*, *extract wisdom*, and *protect ourselves energetically*. Just as proteins remain intact in the gut, so do old emotions and trauma in the psyche.

"Low stomach acid mirrors a soul that has been suppressing its truth—failing to assert, to digest, to transform."

Enzyme Deficiency: Missing the Alchemical Keys

Digestive enzymes are the body's internal alchemists—transforming the physical into usable fuel. When they are depleted, food stagnates and inflammation follows.

Symptoms:

- Fatigue shortly after meals

- Undigested fats in stool

- Skin breakouts or rashes

- Cravings for sugar or carbs

Spiritual Impact:

Enzymes are symbolic of our **capacity to assimilate**—to take in the experiences of life and turn them into embodied wisdom. When enzyme function is low, we may take in too much without properly processing, leading to emotional overflow, confusion, and dependency on external stimulants.

Gas, Bloating, and Irregular Bowel Movements: Inner Chaos

Gas and bloating are often signs of microbial imbalance, poor digestion, or incomplete breakdown of food. Over time, this can lead to **IBS, constipation, or**

loose stools—all indications that the body's rhythm is out of sync.

Spiritual Implications:

- Gut chaos reflects **internal dissonance**

- Constipation can reflect **emotional holding and fear of release**

- Loose stools often symbolize **inability to ground or integrate**

- IBS is a manifestation of a nervous system caught between fight and flight

"The gut is the subconscious mind. When it is inflamed, confused, or dysregulated, so are we."

The Forgotten Compass: Foggy Intuition and Suppressed Instinct

Your gut is your second brain—and the home of your **intuition**, your **instinct**, your **emotional intelligence**. When digestive fire is depleted, this intuitive signal weakens. You may feel:

- Spiritually disconnected

- Chronically fatigued

- Prone to emotional volatility

- Unclear about decisions or boundaries

This isn't just psychological—it's **neurochemical**. Gut bacteria influence serotonin, dopamine, and GABA. The enteric nervous system—embedded in the gut wall—communicates directly with the brain and the heart. When this network is compromised, so is your **inner guidance system**.

🧘 Healing the Fire: Reigniting Digestive and Spiritual Vitality

To restore digestive fire is to **restore trust in oneself**, to **reconnect to rhythm**, to **listen once more to the body's quiet wisdom**.

Practices to Rebuild Digestive Fire:

- **Bitters** before meals to stimulate HCl

- **Enzyme support** (especially lipase, protease, and amylase)

- **Ginger tea**, fennel, cumin, and carminative herbs

- **Mindful eating**: no screens, no rushing, chew thoroughly

- **Cyclical eating**: break from constant surplus (especially after bulking phases)

- **Time to digest**—both food and life

- **Emotional processing**—let go of what you're holding

"Healing digestion is not just about food—it's about **receiving**, **feeling**, and **trusting** again."

D. Gut Flora and the Energetic Body

🌿 The Microbiome as Spiritual Intelligence

Your gut is home to more neurons than your spinal cord. It produces over **90% of your serotonin** — the neurotransmitter most associated with peace, stability, and joy. It shapes your immune system, your metabolism, and even your personality. But more subtly, it regulates how grounded, emotionally regulated, and **spiritually available** you are.

The microbiome is **alive with communication**, adapting constantly to your environment, your thoughts, your food, and your emotional state. In a spiritual sense, it acts as an **intra-dimensional translator**—receiving the impressions of the outer world and offering internal guidance based on energetic balance.

"Your gut flora is your inner choir. When it is in harmony, the song of the soul is clear."

When the Choir Falls into Discord: Dysbiosis, SIBO, Candida

When this microbial harmony is disrupted—by stress, poor diet, antibiotics, overuse of PEDs, or toxic thought patterns—the balance tips. This imbalance is called **dysbiosis**, and it manifests in many modern gut-related conditions like:

- **SIBO (Small Intestinal Bacterial Overgrowth)**

- **Candida overgrowth**

- **Leaky gut (intestinal permeability)**

- **Parasite dominance or fungal imbalances**

Physical Symptoms May Include:
- Bloating, gas, discomfort after meals

- Brain fog, fatigue, or skin eruptions

- Sugar cravings or mood instability

- Immune dysregulation or food intolerances

Spiritual Consequences:
- Foggy or distorted intuition

- Overthinking or emotional reactivity

- Depression or anxiety without clear cause

- Disconnection from body's signals and boundaries

- Hyper-sensitivity to external energy fields (or total numbness)

"Dysbiosis is not just a biological event. It is a breakdown in your capacity to process life clearly and wholly."

🌸 Healthy Flora: Anchoring Emotional and Spiritual Integrity

A thriving microbiome supports:

- **Emotional balance**, through GABA and serotonin production

- **Nervous system regulation**, calming the fight-or-flight response

- **Grounded awareness**, keeping you embodied and present

- **Spiritual discernment**, allowing you to tell resonance from distortion

Much like a forest, the diversity and harmony of your internal ecosystem determines how **resilient** and **responsive** your system is. A well-tended gut is like sacred soil—able to nourish, protect, and regenerate not only the body but the **soul's expression through the body**.

"When the gut is healed, the heart feels safe to open."

🌿 Restoring the Inner Garden: A Protocol of Reverence

Rather than "killing off the bad bugs," healing the microbiome requires an approach of **relationship and respect**. We do not wage war on the gut; we listen, we nurture, we rewild.

Key Practices:

- **Prebiotic fiber** from plants: garlic, leeks, onions, asparagus, dandelion

- **Fermented foods** in moderation: sauerkraut, kimchi, kefir, miso

- **Polyphenols**: berries, green tea, cacao, turmeric

- **Digestive bitters** to support bile flow and enzymatic activity

- **Parasympathetic eating**: slow meals, chewing, gratitude

- **Emotional processing**: journaling, therapy, or plant medicine integration

- **Detoxification**: binders like activated charcoal, chlorella, or zeolite to absorb die-off toxins

- **Time in nature**: exposure to biodiverse environments inoculates the body with resilient bacteria

🧘 Conclusion: You Are a Multitude

To honor the microbiome is to **honor complexity**—to respect the unseen forces that shape who we are and how we move through the world. In bodybuilding, the temptation is often to simplify the body into calories, reps, and aesthetics. But underneath the muscle, the soul speaks in ecosystems, not equations.

True strength arises not just from what we build, but from how deeply we listen to what is already there.

E. Periodization of Feeding – Honoring Digestive Recovery

📅 Sacred Cycles: Periodization of Feeding

The body, like the seasons, thrives on **phases of abundance and restoration**. Below are practical models for incorporating digestive recovery into your lifestyle — whether bulking, prepping, or transitioning.

🌀 1. One-Day Weekly Digestive Break

- **What:** 1 day per week of reduced volume eating — bone broths, smoothies, stewed vegetables, teas, electrolytes

- **Why:** Reduces digestive workload, gives the gut lining time to repair, enhances clarity and sensitivity

- **Spiritual Benefit:** A time of lightness and reflection; mirrors the Sabbath principle — rest as integration

"Give the body one day a week not to grow, but to absorb."

2. 3–4 Weeks of Caloric Cycling

- **What:** Alternate between slight surplus and maintenance every 3–4 weeks

- **Why:** Prevents chronic inflammation, improves insulin sensitivity, allows enzymatic systems to catch up

- **Spiritual Benefit:** Reminds us that **growth is cyclical**, not linear — space is a catalyst, not a threat

This also mimics the lunar rhythm — full moon (abundance), new moon (stillness).

3. Seasonal Rebalancing (Post-Competition)

- **What:** After a show or cut, initiate a **gut repair phase** before rebounding calories too aggressively

- **Key Focus:**

  o Gentle reintroduction of complex carbs

  o Digestive bitters and enzymes

  o Rebuilding the microbiome with pre- and probiotics

- **Why:** Post-prep digestion is fragile; sudden surpluses can cause **gut shock, bloating, water retention**, and mental disorientation

- **Spiritual Benefit:** Aligning with seasonal death and rebirth — competition prep is the winter; rebalancing is spring

"If we don't allow time to digest what we consume — food or experience — we stagnate spiritually."

4. Strategic Reintroduction of Macronutrients

- **What:** Slowly reintroduce **carbs and fats** over 2–3 weeks post-prep, based on energy expenditure

- **Why:** Sharp spikes can overwhelm the pancreas, gallbladder, and microbiota; cause mood crashes, fatigue

- **Spiritual Benefit:** Practicing reverence and patience with food mirrors patience in the unfolding of life

Reintegration is not a punishment — it's a **devotional act of rebuilding communion with the body.**

Digestive Sovereignty as Spiritual Mastery

When we stop forcing food into the system and begin listening for when the system is ready to receive, we regain something far more valuable than calories — **sovereignty.**

We learn to **trust the body again.**

We stop chasing macros and start cultivating wisdom.

And perhaps most importantly — we learn that **muscle grown with respect is stronger**, more enduring, and more spiritually aligned than muscle grown through force.

- Sample timelines for relief:

  - **1-day weekly digestive break** (liquids, broths, lower volume)

- o **3-4 weeks of caloric cycling** between surplus and maintenance

- o Seasonal rebalancing (post-competition: intuitive eating, gut repair phase)

- **Strategic reintroduction** of carbs/fats post-prep to avoid gut shock

"Growth is not linear. Neither is digestion. Periods of stillness allow the fire to burn cleaner."

F. Structuring a Spiritually-Aligned Nutrition Plan

- Eating for nourishment, not punishment

- Practicing **mindful chewing**, parasympathetic eating state, and gratitude

- Prioritizing foods that:

  - o Enhance gut motility (fiber, bitters)

  - o Support enzyme function (papaya, pineapple, fermented foods)

  - o Rebuild the lining (collagen, glutamine, bone broth)

G. Tools to Prevent or Heal Digestive Disorders

- **Digestive enzymes**: lipase, amylase, protease, HCl for heavy meals

- **Herbal antimicrobials**: for early-stage SIBO/candida (berberine, oregano oil, etc.)

- **Probiotics and prebiotics**: targeted strains (like *Lactobacillus* and *Bifido*) post-antibiotic or high PED phases

  - GI Testing when needed (GI-MAP, organic acids, SIBO breath tests)

Chapter 10: Purification and Power – Detoxification as Spiritual Discipline

A. The BOHR effect

The **Bohr effect** describes how **carbon dioxide (CO_2) and pH levels affect hemoglobin's ability to bind and release oxygen**. Specifically:

As CO_2 increases and blood becomes more acidic (lower pH), hemoglobin releases more oxygen to the tissues.

This is normally adaptive. But in the context of **performance enhancing drug (PED) abuse**, it becomes a **double-edged sword**—exacerbating **systemic imbalances** and pushing the body deeper into **stress, hypoxia, and dysfunction.**

🧬 THE BOHR EFFECT: QUICK REVIEW

1. Discovered by Christian Bohr (1904).

2. High CO_2 and low pH (acidic) = more O_2 released from hemoglobin.

3. Low CO_2 and high pH (alkaline) = hemoglobin holds onto O_2.

4. It's a **mechanism of oxygen delivery**, especially during intense exercise or stress.

⚠ HOW PED ABUSE INTERFERES WITH THE BOHR EFFECT

PEDs create **chronic metabolic stress**, often mimicking or exaggerating the conditions that activate the Bohr effect—**but without the recovery phase**, leading to **pathological adaptations**.

1. Anabolic Steroids → Increased Metabolic Demand & Acid Load

- **Effect**: Accelerated muscle mass increases **oxygen consumption** and **lactic acid production**.

- **Interaction**: More CO_2 → more oxygen release... **but tissues are now inflamed, hypoxic, or dysfunctional**.

- **Consequence**: Oxygen is dumped into "toxic" environments—failing to nourish the cells properly.

Spiritual echo: The body is trying to *give*, but the terrain is too toxic to *receive*. A metaphor for burnout and overgiving.

2. Stimulants (e.g., clenbuterol, ephedrine) → Respiratory Alkalosis

- **Effect**: Hyperventilation reduces CO_2 → **less Bohr effect**.

- **Interaction**: Hemoglobin holds onto oxygen → **tissue hypoxia**, especially in the brain and heart.

- **Consequence**: Paradoxical fatigue, anxiety, poor cognition—despite high blood oxygen levels.

Spiritual echo: You are "breathing fast but not breathing deep"—disconnected from the soul's natural rhythm.

3. Human Growth Hormone (HGH) → Organ & Tissue Enlargement

1. **Effect**: Increased tissue mass = increased demand for oxygen.

2. **Interaction**: If vascular and mitochondrial support doesn't keep up, **relative hypoxia** sets in.

3. **Consequence**: More CO_2 buildup → chronic Bohr activation → **overdelivery of O_2**, but to poorly perfused or inflamed areas.

Energetically: Like overfeeding a starving man fast food—nutrients can't integrate.

4. Insulin Misuse → Disrupted Cellular Respiration

- **Effect**: Artificially driven glucose into cells without proper mitochondrial readiness = increased lactate.

- **Interaction**: More acid in bloodstream → stronger Bohr effect → oxygen release.

- **Consequence**: Yet again, tissues aren't ready to use that oxygen, leading to **oxidative stress and cellular damage**.

5. Dehydration & Diuretics → Blood Thickening

- **Effect**: Reduced plasma volume raises blood viscosity and impairs gas exchange.

- **Interaction**: Even with Bohr-mediated O_2 dumping, red blood cells can't reach peripheral tissues effectively.

- **Consequence**: Peripheral hypoxia, cramps, brain fog, and vascular strain.

COGNITIVE & NEUROSPIRITUAL IMPACT

- **Brain** is extremely sensitive to **oxygen tension**.

- PED abuse + altered Bohr dynamics = hypoxia in brain tissue → **cognitive fog, mood swings, emotional dysregulation**.

- Chronic sympathetic dominance (fight-or-flight) keeps CO_2 levels artificially low—**suppressing Bohr effect** when it's actually needed during rest.

- **Poor sleep and glymphatic drainage** further limit oxygenation in cerebral tissue.

Spiritual consequence: Difficulty connecting to intuition, dreams, or higher guidance—brain is underfed even while body is overstimulated.

🔄 VISCERAL CYCLE OF DAMAGE

1. **PEDs increase intensity and metabolic byproducts (CO_2, H^+).**

2. **Bohr effect attempts to compensate by increasing O_2 delivery.**

3. **But compromised vascular, mitochondrial, and detox systems can't integrate O_2 effectively.**

4. **Result = oxidative stress, tissue damage, spiritual disconnection.**

🌀 SPIRITUAL METAPHOR OF THE BOHR EFFECT UNDER STRESS

The Bohr effect is like a wise elder saying:

"Give more oxygen where it's needed most."

PEDs, however, create a state where the body **cries out for oxygen**, but the tissues are too damaged or inflamed to receive it. This mimics the **human experience of overachievement**—striving, pushing, reaching—but **without integration, nourishment, or sacred rest**.

✴ HEALING IMPLICATIONS

- **CO_2 tolerance training** (e.g., Buteyko breathing, nasal breathing, altitude masks).

- **Deep sleep and glymphatic support** → oxygen delivery to brain improves.

- **Mitochondrial support**: magnesium, CoQ10, B vitamins, NAD+.

- **Spiritual recalibration**: practices that **slow down the breath and mind—** breathwork, meditation, floating.

Quick Recap: The Bohr Effect

- The Bohr effect states that **higher CO_2 levels (and lower blood pH)** cause hemoglobin to release more oxygen to tissues.

- Conversely, **low CO_2 (from over-breathing/hyperventilation)** makes hemoglobin hold onto oxygen — causing tissue hypoxia even if blood oxygen looks normal.

- So, CO_2 tolerance = better oxygen delivery.

Breathwork and the Bohr Effect

1. Slower Breathing / CO_2 Retention

- Techniques: **Buteyko method, nasal breathing, box breathing**.

- Effects:

  o Increases CO_2 tolerance.

  o Optimizes hemoglobin's oxygen release to muscles and brain.

  o Improves endurance, recovery, and cognitive clarity.

- **Example**: Athletes who practice nasal breathing during training adapt to higher CO_2 levels, allowing better oxygen unloading in performance states.

2. Breath Holds / Controlled Hypoxia

- Techniques: **Wim Hof method (breath retention after exhalation), pranayama (kumbhaka)**.

- Effects:

  - Temporary hypoxia → spike in CO_2.

  - Strongly drives the Bohr effect → increased oxygen dumping into tissues after the hold.

- Benefits:

  - Stimulates erythropoietin (EPO) → more red blood cells.

  - Enhances mitochondria's efficiency at using oxygen.

3. Diaphragmatic Breathing

- Engaging the diaphragm maximizes alveolar gas exchange.

- More efficient exchange means:

  - Higher baseline CO_2 tolerance.

  - Balanced O_2/CO_2 ratio → steadier pH.

  - More consistent Bohr effect activation under stress.

4. CO_2 Training for Performance

- Breathwork can be applied like strength training for the respiratory system:

  - **Exhale-hold walking/running drills** to elevate CO_2.

  - Improves tolerance to lactic acid during high-intensity work.

  - Muscles receive oxygen more efficiently even under metabolic stress.

🧠 Emotional & Spiritual Layers

- **Calm Breath = Calm Mind**: Slower breathing entrains parasympathetic dominance, reducing emotional volatility (common in PED/stimulant use).

- **CO_2 as a Messenger**: It doesn't just drive oxygen release — it influences neural excitability and vagal tone, linking breath to mood regulation.

- **Breath Holds as Ceremony**: Extended retention pushes awareness inward, enhances clarity, and simulates altered states where the body "trusts" oxygen will arrive.

Practical Breathwork Protocol for Bohr Optimization

1. **Daily CO_2 Tolerance Training**

   o   10–15 min of slow nasal breathing (inhale 4–6 sec, exhale 6–8 sec).

2. **Performance Prep**

   o   2–3 rounds of breath holds (after normal exhale) before training to condition tolerance.

3. **Recovery / Sleep**

   o   Box breathing (4-4-4-4) or extended exhalation breathing (inhale 4, exhale 8) before bed.

4. **Spiritual Practice**

   o   Combine retention + visualization to deepen meditation and nervous system release.

In short: **Breathwork optimizes the Bohr effect by raising CO_2 tolerance, stabilizing pH, and improving oxygen delivery where it's most needed** — brain, heart, and working muscles.

Performance enhancing drugs (PEDs)—including anabolic steroids, growth hormone, insulin, stimulants, and nootropics—have complex and often poorly understood effects on the lymphatic and glymphatic systems. While most research focuses on muscular, cardiovascular, and endocrine outcomes, the subtle and systemic nature of these clearance and detox systems means they are deeply affected over time. Below is a breakdown of how PEDs may affect these systems across physical, emotional, biochemical, and spiritual dimensions.

THE GLYMPHATIC SYSTEM

<u>Overview:</u>

The glymphatic system is the brain's waste clearance mechanism, primarily active during deep sleep. It clears metabolic byproducts, inflammatory proteins, and even toxins like amyloid beta—linked to Alzheimer's.

1. Biochemical Effects of PEDs on the Glymphatic System

- **Sleep disruption** (especially from stimulants, testosterone, or Trenbolone) reduces glymphatic activity.

- **Corticosteroids or chronic sympathetic activation** can constrict cerebrovascular flow, reducing glymphatic fluid exchange.

- **Increased oxidative stress and neuroinflammation**, often seen with long-term PED use, impairs glymphatic efficiency.

- **Dehydration** from diuretics or cutting agents thickens CSF and interstitial fluids, slowing clearance.

2. Physical Implications

- **Cognitive fog**, poor memory consolidation, and slower recovery from neural fatigue.

- **Higher risk of neurodegenerative disease** over time due to accumulation of tau and amyloid proteins.

- **Headaches, pressure sensations**, or signs of neuroinflammation.

3. Emotional Implications

- Emotional dysregulation from PED-induced poor sleep leads to:

- Mood swings

- Irritability

- Lower emotional resilience

- Anxiety and overstimulation often result when the brain cannot effectively "clean house."

4. Spiritual Implications

- A "clogged" glymphatic system can block access to **higher states of awareness** that depend on deep sleep and dream integration.

- Users may feel **disconnected from their intuition or inner knowing**.

- Artificial stimulation (stimulants, nootropics) can lead to spiritual bypassing—**mistaking ego-driven productivity for spiritual alignment**.

THE LYMPHATIC SYSTEM

Overview:

The lymphatic system is responsible for detoxification, immune surveillance, fluid balance, and absorption of fats. It works closely with the cardiovascular and immune systems.

1. Biochemical Effects of PEDs on the Lymphatic System

- **Anabolic steroids** can increase lymphocyte count initially but **impair immune function long-term**, leading to sluggish lymph drainage and toxic accumulation.

- **Exogenous hormones** and **synthetic agents** often cause **systemic inflammation**, burdening lymphatic flow.

- **Growth hormone and insulin misuse** can enlarge organs and tissues (acromegaly), which may compress lymphatic vessels.

2. Physical Implications

- **Lymphatic congestion** presents as:

  o Puffiness

  o Water retention

  o Swollen glands

  o Fatigue

- Weakened immune defense leads to **increased susceptibility to infections and slow healing**.

- Over time, this can evolve into **chronic inflammation, autoimmune tendencies**, and even **lymphatic cancers**.

3. Emotional Implications

- Chronic lymph stagnation is associated with:

  o Emotional heaviness

  o Anger held in the tissues

  o A sense of being stuck or burdened

- PED users may feel emotionally volatile or numbed, as the body can no longer regulate inflammatory signals properly.

4. Spiritual Implications

- The lymphatic system plays a crucial role in **emotional and energetic detoxification**.

- A congested lymphatic system mirrors a **blocked or repressed emotional body**, often seen in those avoiding vulnerability or grief.

- Spiritually, this can feel like:

  o **Disconnection from Source**

  o **Inability to feel authentic joy or compassion**

  o **Energetic rigidity or armor**

🔋 COMPOUNDING FACTORS

1. **Stacking PEDs** amplifies systemic stress—e.g., using Tren + HGH + Stimulants creates a perfect storm for neurotoxic buildup and lymphatic inflammation.

2. **Lack of recovery protocols** (sleep, sauna, lymphatic drainage, fasting) worsens long-term damage.

3. **Liver and kidney strain** from PEDs reduces toxin clearance, forcing the lymphatic system to pick up the slack.

✴ HEALING AND RESTORATION

Approach	Impact
Manual lymphatic drainage	Supports detox and reduces water retention.
Deep sleep enhancement (melatonin, glycine, breathwork)	Activates glymphatic system.
Emotional processing (somatic therapy, breathwork)	Clears stuck emotions tied to lymphatic congestion.

Spiritual alignment (fasting, nature immersion, plant medicine)	Reconnects intuition and clears egoic residue from PEDs.
Nervous system repair (adaptogens, magnesium, float therapy)	Calms sympathetic dominance, improving fluid flow.

🔑 Summary

System	PED Effects	Consequences
Glymphatic	Sleep disruption, inflammation, oxidative stress	Cognitive decline, emotional instability, spiritual numbness
Lymphatic	Hormonal imbalance, inflammation, immune dysfunction	Puffiness, chronic fatigue, emotional stagnation, disconnection

PEDs provide short-term power at the cost of **long-term flow**. They amplify **egoic will** while often suppressing **organic intelligence**. Over time, this imbalance leads to toxic buildup—physical, emotional, and spiritual.

If you're using or considering PEDs, integrating **detox, emotional awareness, and spiritual grounding** is crucial to preserve wholeness and prevent decay beneath the surface.

Toxins in the Modern Iron Temple

The Hidden Burden: Endocrine Disruptors & Heavy Metals as Silent Saboteurs

In the modern world, we are exposed daily to a vast array of chemicals that **mimic, disrupt, or suppress natural hormonal rhythms**. These substances, often invisible, insidiously interfere with our biochemistry — hijacking our physiology, muting our emotions, and even dulling our spiritual perception.

Their impact is not limited to the physical body. These agents carry **an energetic weight** — a kind of density that dampens clarity, intuition, and our connection to the subtle currents of life. True purification of the body is not just about detoxifying organs; it's about **liberating the inner signal** — restoring access to the unfiltered intelligence of the self.

🧬 Biochemical and Physical Consequences

1. Food Sources

Glyphosate (RoundUp), pesticides, artificial sweeteners (e.g., aspartame, sucralose):

These are potent **xenoestrogens** and **neurotoxins** that:

- Disrupt the gut microbiome, leading to increased permeability ("leaky gut")

- Mimic estrogen, creating hormonal imbalance (testosterone suppression, PCOS, estrogen dominance)

- Burden the liver, impairing detox pathways (Phase I/II)

- Damage mitochondrial function (fatigue, slowed recovery)

- Alter insulin sensitivity, impacting nutrient partitioning and fat storage

Physical Symptoms:

- Fat gain in stubborn areas (lower abs, thighs, chest)

- Brain fog, fatigue, sleep disturbances

- Digestive issues (bloating, irregular bowel movements)

- Skin conditions (acne, eczema)

- Plateaus in muscle growth despite proper training and diet

2. Water Contaminants

<u>Fluoride, chlorine, PFAS (forever chemicals):</u>

- Fluoride is a known **pineal gland calcifier**, limiting melatonin production and spiritual perception

- PFAS (found in nonstick pans, plastics, and water) bioaccumulate in fat and are linked to **thyroid disruption**

- Chlorine and chloramine affect gut flora and suppress immune function

<u>Biochemical Impact:</u>

- Lowered testosterone and fertility

- Disrupted circadian rhythm

- Elevated inflammation markers (CRP, homocysteine)

- Impaired metabolic detoxification (especially glucuronidation and sulfation)

<u>Physical Symptoms:</u>

- Anxiety, restlessness, poor sleep quality

- Brain fog, depressive states

- Adrenal and thyroid dysfunction (fatigue, cold intolerance, weight gain)

3. Airborne Contaminants

Urban smog, VOCs (from paint, plastics, perfumes), mold spores:

- VOCs (Volatile Organic Compounds) interfere with **neurotransmitter balance** (especially dopamine and serotonin)

- Mold produces **mycotoxins** that can impair mitochondrial ATP production

- Polluted air affects **oxygen uptake** → limiting endurance, recovery, and cognitive sharpness

Biochemical & Physical Symptoms:

- Low-grade systemic inflammation

- Persistent fatigue despite rest

- Hormonal imbalances (especially cortisol and thyroid)

- Autoimmune triggers (molecular mimicry)

💜 Emotional Impact: Numbness, Dysregulation, and Disconnect

These endocrine disruptors not only clog the body's filtration systems — they also **distort the emotional body**. The gut-brain axis is heavily influenced by chemical burden. When the **gut is inflamed and the liver is overwhelmed**, emotional regulation suffers.

Common emotional manifestations include:

- Irritability, short temper, emotional reactivity

- Inability to feel joy or peace consistently

- Emotional numbness and disconnection

- Heightened stress response (even in safe environments)

- Loss of motivation or discipline (dopamine pathway disruption)

Over time, this creates **emotional dissociation** from the body, and we begin to relate to it like a machine — something to control, manipulate, or shame — rather than a sacred vessel of intuition and feeling.

🪷 Spiritual Consequences: Dimmed Awareness and Suppressed Intuition

The spiritual implications are subtle, but deeply profound:

- **Pineal Gland Calcification:** Fluoride and heavy metals dull the very gland associated with **vision, dreams, inner knowing, and the connection to Source.**

- **Energetic Congestion**: Toxins are not just matter — they hold frequency. When they accumulate, they lower the body's overall **vibratory tone**, creating stagnation in the energy body and auric field.

- **Loss of Sensitivity**: Subtle perceptions — emotional cues, intuitive hits, spiritual downloads — become harder to detect. We lose our **inner compass**.

- **Spiritual Exhaustion**: Just as the body tires under chemical burden, so too does the **spirit grow weary** when trapped in a vessel it cannot fully express through.

"Toxins create static. Detoxification clears the signal so Spirit can speak through us — clearly, cleanly, and consistently."

🌿 The Path Forward: Conscious Detoxification

- **Install a reverse osmosis water filter** and remineralize

- **Buy organic or local produce** to minimize pesticide load

- **Limit exposure to plastic and nonstick cookware**

- **Sweat regularly**: sauna, cardio, and breathwork

- **Use binders** (activated charcoal, zeolite) and liver support herbs (milk thistle, dandelion)

- **Mold mitigation**: HEPA filters, regular cleaning, test your home if symptoms persist

- **Energetic detox**: use breathwork, prayer, ceremony, or plant medicines to clear stagnation from the energetic body

🧘 Integration Is the Goal

Detoxification is not just about elimination — it's about **recalibration**. It's about returning the body to its role as a clear instrument of the soul — vibrant, receptive, and sovereign.

The cleaner the system, the louder the signal. The lighter the body, the deeper the presence. In this clarity, we don't just build physiques — **we become channels**.

The Shadow Side of Supplementation: Red Flags in the Wellness Industry

In a culture obsessed with peak performance, enhancement, and transformation, supplements have become a modern sacrament. Powdered nutrition, nootropics, SARMs, and muscle-building aids are often consumed daily without pause — rarely questioned, seldom respected.

Yet beneath the glossy packaging and influencer endorsements lies a darker truth: **many supplements are laced with synthetic chemicals, hidden contaminants, and energetically dead materials.** When we ingest these daily, we aren't just compromising our physical health — we are dulling our intuition, disrupting our biochemistry, and confusing our spiritual intelligence.

🧬 Biochemical & Physical Impacts

1. Synthetic Fillers:

Common examples: Magnesium stearate, titanium dioxide, silicon dioxide, talc

These agents are often used to increase shelf life, improve flow during manufacturing, or make tablets look uniform — but they offer **zero nutritional value** and may impair absorption.

Biochemical/Physical Effects:

- **Titanium dioxide** has been classified as a potential **carcinogen** and can cause **gut inflammation**

- **Magnesium stearate** can **inhibit nutrient absorption**, especially in sensitive individuals

- May irritate the GI lining and **disrupt the gut microbiome**

Symptoms to watch for:

- Bloating, irregular stools, stomach discomfort

- Nutrient deficiencies despite supplementation

- Headaches or fatigue after taking supplements

2. Artificial Sweeteners & Dyes:

Common examples: Aspartame, sucralose, acesulfame potassium, Red 40, Yellow 5

These compounds are used to mask poor flavor or make powders more visually appealing — especially in **mass-market pre-workouts, fat burners, flavored proteins, and hydration mixes**.

Biochemical Effects:

- Disrupt gut flora, promoting **dysbiosis, candida, and SIBO**

- Aspartame and sucralose can **alter glucose metabolism and insulin response**

- Artificial dyes have been linked to **neurological changes** and **hyperactivity**, especially in children

Symptoms to watch for:

- Brain fog, anxiety, or mood instability

- Sugar cravings, blood sugar crashes

- Chronic bloating or digestive discomfort

- Poor recovery and inconsistent energy

3. Contaminants in Low-Quality Products:

Frequent offenders:

- **Whey proteins** from cows raised on GMO feed and antibiotics

- **SARMs** (often mislabeled, contaminated, or mixed with prohormones or steroids)

- **Nootropics** with unknown Chinese synthetics, trace heavy metals, or illegal analogs

Physical & Biochemical Risks:

- Liver and kidney stress from unknown chemical cocktails

- Endocrine disruption from hidden androgens or estrogens

- Adrenal burnout from stimulant-laced formulas

- Toxic load accumulation that overwhelms detox organs

Symptoms to watch for:

- Hormonal imbalances (acne, hair loss, libido changes)

- Elevated liver enzymes or kidney markers on bloodwork

- Anxiety, insomnia, or stimulant dependence

- Sudden mood changes or emotional instability

💜 Emotional & Psychological Impact

When we consume impure, synthetic, or deceptive products — especially over time — the effects extend beyond biology.

Energetic & Emotional Impacts:

- **Loss of trust in one's body:** If results are inconsistent or side effects unpredictable, it creates confusion and insecurity about the body's feedback

- **Addictive behaviors:** Especially with SARMs, fat burners, or pre-workouts — reliance on external substances to *feel worthy*, *motivated*, or *in control*

- **Emotional suppression:** Some ingredients (stimulants, synthetic nootropics) override natural emotional processing, keeping us in a high-strung sympathetic state

"When we consistently override the body's whispers with synthetic stimulation, we lose access to its deeper wisdom."

🧠 Spiritual Consequences

- **Distorted Relationship with Nature:** Supplements should be allies. When filled with synthetics, they reflect a mindset of *domination over nature* instead of *partnership with it.*

- **Pollution of the Temple:** The body is the vessel of spirit. Polluting it with toxins for the sake of quick gains, faster recovery, or "hacking" our biology sends a subconscious signal: *my natural state is not enough.*

- **Suppressed Intuition:** Poor gut health → foggy mind → lost clarity. When the gut is inflamed and energetically burdened, it becomes harder to hear **spiritual nudges**, make clean decisions, or trust instinct.

Karmic Entanglement: Supporting companies that profit from deception or low-quality, harmful ingredients contributes to collective harm. We become spiritually entangled in **systems that exploit human vitality.**

⚠ How to Protect Yourself

<u>Choose Clean, Conscious Supplementation:</u>

- Look for **third-party testing** (NSF, Informed Choice, USP, or BSCG certified)

- Avoid products with long chemical names or artificial colors/sweeteners

- Choose **whole-food-based supplements** wherever possible

- Prioritize **formulations designed by functional medicine practitioners** or ethically aligned brands

- Always **cycle off** high-stimulant products to recalibrate sensitivity

<u>Red Flags Checklist:</u>

- Ingredients you can't pronounce

- Proprietary blends without full breakdowns

- Unrealistic claims ("Lose 10 lbs in 10 days")

- No clear sourcing or testing data

- Cheap prices that seem too good to be true

🧘 A. Spiritual Approach to Supplementation

Supplements should **amplify what is already working** in the body — not replace discipline, nourishment, or intuition.

Before taking anything new, ask:

- *What is the deeper need I m trying to meet?"*

- *Do I feel empowered or dependent using this?"*

- *Is this enhancing my connection to my body or overriding it?"*

The right supplements act like allies — quiet support on the path of integration. The wrong ones act like tyrants — demanding obedience while slowly eroding sovereignty.

B. The Adrenal Trap – Overstimulated, Under-souled

- Chronic pre-workouts, caffeine, stimulants = adrenal burnout

- Short-term gain, long-term crash: cortisol dysregulation, thyroid slowdown, mood instability

- Energetically: detaches consciousness from the parasympathetic "receiving" state, leading to **spiritual disconnection and nervous system exhaustion**

"In seeking constant performance, we forget how to *receive* life."

C. Signs You Need a Detox (Physical, Emotional, Spiritual)

- Brain fog, fatigue, poor recovery, skin issues

- Short temper, anxiety, spiritual numbness

- Digestive stagnation or inflammation

- Disconnection from breath, silence, or spiritual practices

- Obsession with stimulation (phones, caffeine, mirrors, lifting)

D. Foundational Detox Protocols for Bodybuilders

<u>Daily Practices:</u>

- Morning hydration with minerals (Himalayan salt, lemon)

- Sweat therapy: sauna 3–5x/week

- Liver support: milk thistle, dandelion root, NAC, castor oil packs

- Intermittent fasting or digestive rest periods

- Tongue scraping, dry brushing, lymphatic movement (walking, rebounding)

- Mold/mycotoxin binders: activated charcoal, bentonite clay, zeolite

<u>Organ-Specific Detox Support:</u>

- **Liver**: bitters, choline, TUDCA, beetroot

- **Kidneys**: nettle tea, dandelion leaf, cranberry

- **Colon**: magnesium citrate, aloe vera, colon hydrotherapy (used wisely)

- **Brain**: magnesium threonate, lion's mane, meditation

E. Sauna, Infrared sauna, Cold Plunge, Cryotherapy and Red Light Therapy (Photobiomodulation) for health and optimal recovery.

🜄 1. TRADITIONAL SAUNA (Dry or Steam)

Heat Stress | Detoxification | Hormetic Adaptation

☑ <u>Best Used When:</u>

- You need **cardiovascular conditioning** without physical strain.

- Detoxing from PEDs, heavy metals, or synthetic substances.

- Enhancing growth hormone post-exercise.

- **Mental clarity** or breaking emotional stagnation.

- To promote **parasympathetic rebound** after intense sympathetic states (e.g., high stress or training).

Mental/Emotional:

- Heat helps release **stored trauma**, especially grief and frustration.

- Meditative states and visions often arise in deep sweat—sacred purification.

Optimal Timing:

- **Post-workout** (20–30 min).

- **Fasted state** (for fat loss or deep detox).

- Not ideal right before bed due to cortisol spike unless followed by a cool shower.

2. INFRARED SAUNA

Cellular Detox | Mitochondrial Activation | Soft Tissue Recovery

Best Used When:

- You need **deeper penetration** into muscles, fascia, and organs.

- You're experiencing **chronic fatigue, autoimmune issues, or toxic accumulation**.

- During **spiritual healing or emotional release** work.

Mental/Emotional:

- Gentle, enveloping heat softens defensive tension held in the body.

- Excellent for **vagal toning** and processing suppressed emotions.

⏱ Optimal Timing:

- **Morning or early afternoon**, especially before meditation or journaling.

- 20–45 minutes, hydration critical before and after.

🧊 3. ICE BATH / COLD PLUNGE

Nervous System Reset | Inflammation Control | Mental Fortitude

✅ Best Used When:

- You need to **reduce inflammation** or soreness rapidly.

- Regulating overstimulated emotions, anxiety, or panic.

- Building **dopamine resilience** and discipline.

- Enhancing **alertness, focus, and willpower**.

🧠 Mental/Emotional:

- Initiates a **state of surrender** to intensity—forces present-moment awareness.

- Helps process fear, resistance, and self-doubt.

- Can feel like a **rebirth ritual** when done with intention.

⏱ Optimal Timing:

- **Morning** for alertness and focus.

- **Post-workout** ONLY if you're not trying to build muscle (can blunt hypertrophy).

- 2–5 min ideal; breathing control is key.

❄ 4. CRYOTHERAPY

Localized or Full-Body Cold | Recovery | Dopamine & Norepinephrine Boost

☑ Best Used When:

- Need **inflammation control** without water immersion (e.g., after surgery or injury).

- You want the **mental benefits of cold** with less emotional intensity than ice baths.

- You're traveling or need a **fast 3-minute recovery tool**.

🧠 Mental/Emotional:

- Boosts resilience and mood, but often feels more clinical and less soul-revealing than ice baths.

- Enhances **neuroplasticity and rewiring patterns** with consistent use.

⏱ Optimal Timing:

- **Pre-workout** (if needing stimulation).

- **Midday dopamine boost** or after high cognitive load.

⬤ 5. RED LIGHT THERAPY (Photobiomodulation)

Cellular Healing | Mitochondrial Support | Hormonal Regulation

☑ Best Used When:

- You're recovering from injury, skin damage, or inflammation.

- For **testosterone and thyroid optimization** (red light on testes/neck).

- For improving **mood, circadian rhythm, and skin health**.

- As part of **trauma recovery** (targets mitochondria = somatic healing).

Mental/Emotional:

- Deeply soothing, especially to those who feel energetically cold or depleted.

- Can support **inner child work** and **self-worth repair**, as it brings warmth to cells symbolically and physically.

⏱ Optimal Timing:

- **Morning or late afternoon** (stimulates circadian light receptors).

- 5–20 minutes per session.

- Best on **bare skin**, no sunscreen or lotions.

🔁 INTEGRATION STRATEGY

🔄 Daily Wellness Flow (Example)

Time	Modality	Purpose
Morning	Ice bath or Cryotherapy	Dopamine, discipline, nervous system priming
Late AM	Red light therapy	Hormonal tune-up, circadian light mimic
Post-workout	Sauna (Traditional or Infrared)	Detox, parasympathetic rebound
Evening (Optional)	Infrared sauna + meditation	Deep tissue healing + emotional processing

✴ SPIRITUAL SYNTHESIS

Modality	Spiritual Archetype	Shadow it Reveals	Soul Lesson
Sauna	Purifier / Phoenix	Suppressed anger, internal chaos	Surrender to transformation
Infrared Sauna	Womb / Healer	Toxic buildup, slow decay	Softening, release
Ice Bath	Warrior / Initiate	Fear, resistance, avoidance	Presence, courage
Cryotherapy	Alchemist	Numbness, detachment	Precision, clarity
Red Light	Nurturer / Sun God	Deficiency, depletion	Worthiness to receive vitality

🌿 E. Plant Medicines for Deep Detox and Alignment

When toxins accumulate not only in the body, but in the **emotional and spiritual layers**, a deeper purge is often needed. Here, **sacred entheogens** offer profound tools for full-spectrum purification and re-alignment. These medicines are the most powerful in the world and need to be treated with reverence. Each medicine requires an assessment with a professional practitioner and a full commitment to the healing process.

1. Kambo (Frog medicine – Amazonian):

- Immediate physical purge: bile, mucus, trauma, heavy metals

- Clears energetic stagnation from liver, blood, lymph

- "Warrior cleanse" that humbles and clears lower chakras

- Requires assessment and certain restrictions apply

2. Iboga (West African root bark):

- Nervous system reset, deep trauma excavation

  - Detoxifies soul from addiction, patterns, ego distortions

  - Brings confrontation and clarity through ancestral wisdom

  - Can be micro dosed daily or will need to set aside one week and extensive preparation for a flood dose.

3. Ayahuasca (Amazonian vine + leaf brew):

- Emotional catharsis, cellular-level cleansing

- Access to unconscious trauma and psychic blockages

- Often addresses core of illness, not just symptoms

- Will require a special diet for two weeks and a 2-3 day immersion process

4. Bufo Alvarius (5-MeO-DMT):

- Rapid ego dissolution

- Clears psycho-spiritual "residue" built up from chronic attachment to identity

- Merges the self back into source, often used after other detox pathways

- Requires mental preparation and proper vetting to ensure safety and optimal outcome

"When the body is clean, the soul speaks louder. When the mind is quiet, the Spirit remembers."

F. Integration is the Key

- Detox is **not just removal**; it's a **return to alignment**

- Post-detox nourishment = whole foods, gentle movement, deep rest

- Reflective journaling, breath-work, stillness to capture the *spiritual messages* of the purge

Chapter 11: PEPTIDES

Peptides are essentially **short chains of amino acids**—the same building blocks that make up proteins—**designed by nature (and now bioengineers) to carry messages inside your body**.

Think of them as **cellular text messages** that tell your tissues *what to do, when to do it, and how intensely* to respond.

Whereas **proteins** can be thousands of amino acids long, **peptides are usually 2–50 amino acids**, which makes them small enough to act **quickly, specifically, and with fewer side effects** than many drugs.

🧬 WHAT PEPTIDES ARE

- **Naturally occurring:** Your body already makes hundreds of peptides—insulin, oxytocin, endorphins, and growth hormone–releasing peptides are examples.

- **Signaling molecules:** They bind to **specific receptors** on cell membranes, triggering cascades of events that change how a cell behaves.

- **Customizable tools:** Scientists can design synthetic peptides to **mimic or enhance** natural signals, or even block harmful ones.

⚙ HOW PEPTIDES WORK IN THE BODY

1. Targeted Signaling

- Each peptide has a **lock-and-key relationship** with a specific receptor.

- When it binds, it can:

  - Activate growth or repair pathways.

  - Reduce inflammation.

  - Promote neuroplasticity.

  - Adjust hormonal balance.

2. Tissue-Specific Action

- Many peptides are selective to certain tissues (brain, skin, gut, muscle).

- This means **fewer systemic side effects** than most drugs.

3. Short Lifespan

- Peptides are quickly broken down by enzymes—this allows for **precise dosing** and reduces long-term accumulation risks.

🌱 SPIRITUAL & EMOTIONAL HEALING DIMENSIONS

- **Restoring flow:** Chronic illness, injury, or inflammation can create emotional heaviness and energetic stagnation. Peptides often help clear the *physical bottlenecks*, allowing emotional and spiritual processes to move forward.

- **Neurochemistry & consciousness:** By stabilizing neurotransmitters and improving brain oxygenation, peptides can help re-open access to intuition, creativity, and meditative depth.

- **Embodiment**: Physical recovery enhances the ability to inhabit your body fully, which deepens emotional awareness and spiritual grounding.

- **Trauma repair**: Neuro-regenerative peptides can make it easier to process trauma without being stuck in the biochemical imprints of the past.

WHY PEPTIDES ARE DIFFERENT FROM TRADITIONAL DRUGS

Peptides	Traditional Drugs
Mimic natural body signals	Often foreign chemical compounds
Target specific receptors	Often broad-spectrum effects
Shorter action, more precise	Can linger and disrupt other systems
Can support *restoration*	Often only *manage symptoms*

LIMITATIONS & CONSIDERATIONS

- **Not a magic fix** – Without nutrition, movement, and stress work, benefits are limited.

- **Purity matters** – Low-quality peptides can contain contaminants.

- **Regulatory status** – Many are "research use only" in some countries.

- **Overuse** – Excess stimulation can cause receptor desensitization.

By the time this book is released, there will be a dozen new peptides in the pipeline getting ready to hit the Compounding pharmacies. This is a general overview of the most popular peptides in circulation as of August 2025. When choosing to work with peptides you must find a trusted source as impure peptides can wreak havoc on your immune system and cause the very problems that you are trying to heal.

IMMUNE MODULATION & SYSTEMIC REPAIR

Thymosin Alpha 1 (Tα1)

- Enhances **T-cell** and **NK cell** function.

- Immune modulation—used in chronic infections, cancer, and autoimmunity.

- May improve **vaccine response** and reduce inflammation.

Thymosin Beta 4 (Tβ4)

- Promotes **tissue regeneration**, angiogenesis, and wound healing.

- Reduces **fibrosis** and inflammation.

- Aids in **cardiac and muscle repair**, including post-MI recovery.

LL-37

- Antimicrobial peptide: fights **bacterial, viral, and fungal** infections.

- Reduces biofilm formation and promotes **immune homeostasis**.

- Used in **chronic infections**, Lyme, and gut inflammation.

REGENERATION, LONGEVITY & REPAIR

Pentadecapeptide (BPC-157)

- **"Body Protecting Compound"**: accelerates healing in gut, tendon, muscle, nerve.

- Anti-inflammatory and cytoprotective.

- Highly synergistic with TB-500 for systemic repair.

Epithalon

- Pineal peptide that **extends telomere length**.

- Balances melatonin cycles, improves sleep and longevity.

- May reduce **cancer risk** and enhance DNA repair.

SS-31 (Elamipretide)
- Mitochondrial-targeted peptide—protects and restores mitochondrial function.

- Reduces **ROS**, improves energy output, cardiac and neuroprotection.

- Used in **mitochondrial diseases**, neurodegeneration, and anti-aging.

GHK-Cu
- Copper peptide for **skin repair, hair growth, and inflammation** modulation.

- Enhances **collagen synthesis**, angiogenesis, and DNA repair.

- Also regulates genes linked to **stem cell activation and anti-aging**.

🧠 COGNITION, MOOD & NEUROPLASTICITY

DSIP (Delta Sleep-Inducing Peptide)
- Enhances **deep (delta wave) sleep**, especially in insomnia or PTSD.

- May stabilize circadian rhythms and regulate cortisol.

- Reduces physical/mental stress and **improves recovery**.

Semax
- Nootropic with neuroprotective, anti-anxiety, and mood-stabilizing effects.

- Enhances **BDNF**, memory, and learning.

- Common in **neurorehab** and stress-related burnout.

Selank

- Anxiolytic and anti-inflammatory with **no sedative effect**.

- Modulates **dopamine and serotonin**, supports emotional balance.

- Cognitive enhancement without overstimulation.

Dihexa

- Powerful neurogenic peptide derived from angiotensin IV.

- Enhances **synaptogenesis and brain connectivity**.

- Potential for **Alzheimer's, TBI, and cognitive enhancement**.

🔶 GROWTH & HORMONE REGULATION

IGF-1 LR3

- Potent analog of IGF-1 with **extended half-life**.

- Promotes **muscle growth, fat loss, cellular repair**.

- Used in physique optimization and **tissue regeneration**.

Sermorelin

- GHRH analog: stimulates **natural GH release**.

- Shorter acting, more natural GH pulse.

- Good for **anti-aging and mild GH deficiencies**.

CJC-1295 (w/ or w/o DAC)

- GHRH analog with longer half-life than Sermorelin.

- Sustained GH elevation = better muscle growth, recovery, sleep.

- Often stacked with Ipamorelin or Ibutamoren.

Ibutamoren (MK-677)

- GH secretagogue mimicking ghrelin.

- Increases **GH and IGF-1** significantly—oral use.

- Promotes **muscle gain, fat loss**, and deeper sleep.

Tesamorelin

- GHRH analog FDA-approved for **HIV-associated lipodystrophy**.

- Reduces **visceral fat** while maintaining muscle.

- May improve insulin sensitivity and cognitive function.

🧬 METABOLIC & MITOCHONDRIAL MODULATION

MOTS-c

- Mitochondrial-encoded peptide regulating **metabolism and insulin sensitivity**.

- Enhances **fat oxidation**, exercise capacity, and metabolic flexibility.

- May mimic fasting benefits and promote **healthy aging**.

ARA-290 (Cibinetide)

- Erythropoietin derivative for **neuropathic pain**, inflammation, and vascular repair.

- Promotes healing of **small nerve fibers** and improves **insulin sensitivity**.

- Used in diabetes, neuropathy, and **autoimmune syndromes**.

Slu-pp-332

- Novel peptide showing promise in **fat loss** via **β3-adrenergic receptor activation**.

- May act as a **non-stimulant metabolic enhancer**.

- Still in experimental phases.

🧠 SUMMARY TABLE BY FUNCTION

Peptide	Primary Benefits
Thymosin Alpha 1	Immune modulation, infection defense
Thymosin Beta 4	Tissue repair, inflammation control
BPC-157	Gut, nerve, tendon healing
Epithalon	Telomere lengthening, longevity
SS-31	Mitochondrial protection
GHK-Cu	Skin, hair, anti-aging
DSIP	Deep sleep, cortisol balance
Semax	Cognitive enhancement, mood
Selank	Anxiety reduction, neuroprotection
Dihexa	Brain regeneration, memory
IGF-1 LR3	Muscle growth, recovery
Sermorelin	GH pulse stimulation
Ibutamoren	GH/IGF-1 increase, sleep
CJC-1295	GH stimulation (long-acting)
Tesamorelin	Visceral fat loss, metabolism
MOTS-C	Metabolic resilience, endurance
-ARA 290	Nerve healing, inflammation
LL-37	Antimicrobial, immune modulation
Slu-pp-332	Fat loss, metabolic activation (early research)

GLP-1 Peptides

GLP-1 peptides (Glucagon-Like Peptide-1 receptor agonists) are a class of drugs/peptides used for **blood sugar regulation, weight loss, and metabolic optimization**. They mimic the action of

the naturally occurring hormone **GLP-1**, which is released from the gut in response to food and has multiple beneficial effects on **metabolism and appetite**.

🧬 HOW GLP-1 PEPTIDES WORK

GLP-1 receptor agonists exert their effects through **multiple metabolic pathways**:

🧬 PRIMARY MECHANISMS:

1. **Enhance Insulin Secretion**

   o Stimulates insulin release in a glucose-dependent manner (only when blood sugar is elevated).

2. **Suppress Glucagon Secretion**

   o Prevents the liver from releasing too much glucose.

3. **Slow Gastric Emptying**

   o Makes you feel fuller longer, reducing appetite.

4. **Act on the Brain**

   o Suppresses hunger signals via the hypothalamus.

5. **Improve Beta-Cell Function**

   o May preserve or improve insulin-producing pancreatic cells.

6. **Promote Weight Loss**

  o   Reduced food intake and slower digestion → caloric deficit.

COMMON GLP-1 PEPTIDES

Peptide	Brand Name	Half-life	Notes
Liraglutide	Victoza, Saxenda	~13 hours	Daily injection
Semaglutide	Ozempic, Wegovy, Rybelsus (oral)	~7 days	Weekly dosing
Dulaglutide	Trulicity	~5 days	Weekly injection
Exenatide	Byetta (short), Bydureon (long)	~2.4–7 days	Contains **Exendin-4**
Tirzepatide	Mounjaro	~5 days	GLP-1 + GIP dual agonist

⚠ EXENDIN-4: WHAT IT IS & WHY IT CAN BE DANGEROUS

Exendin-4 is a synthetic peptide originally derived from **Gila monster venom**. It was the foundation of the first GLP-1 mimetic: **Exenatide (Byetta and Bydureon)**.

BIOLOGICAL PROFILE OF EXENDIN-4

- Mimics GLP-1, but has **44 amino acids**, whereas human GLP-1 has 30.

- It binds to the **GLP-1 receptor**, but **is not identical to human GLP-1**.

- It is **resistant to DPP-4 breakdown**, giving it a longer half-life.

RISKS & CONCERNS WITH EXENDIN-4–BASED DRUGS

1. **Higher Immunogenicity**

    o   Being **non-human**, exendin-4 can provoke immune reactions.

o Anti-drug antibodies may develop, decreasing effectiveness and increasing inflammation.

2. **Pancreatitis & Pancreatic Cancer Risk**

   o Early studies raised concerns that exendin-4 could overstimulate pancreatic cells, leading to inflammation.

   o Though evidence is inconclusive, **GLP-1 analogs with exendin-4 show a stronger link** than human-based analogs like semaglutide.

3. **Gastrointestinal Side Effects**

   o Nausea, vomiting, and delayed gastric emptying are more pronounced.

   o Risk of **gastroparesis** may be higher with exendin-4 compounds.

4. **Cross-Reactivity or Toxicity**

   o Since it originates from a venom protein, its **long-term systemic safety** is less established.

☑ SAFER ALTERNATIVES TO EXENDIN-4–BASED GLP-1 AGONISTS

Opt for **human-based GLP-1 analogs**:

- **Semaglutide (Ozempic, Wegovy)** — highly effective, less immunogenic.

- **Liraglutide (Victoza)** — older but well-studied.

- **Tirzepatide (Mounjaro)** — newer dual-action (GLP-1 + GIP), excellent results in weight loss and insulin sensitivity.

🧘 SPIRITUAL / LONG-TERM CONSIDERATIONS

1. GLP-1 agonists **numb hunger**, which can be a blessing short-term—but long-term use may **disconnect people from intuitive eating and emotional awareness**.

2. **Appetite is a spiritual compass**; numbing it without addressing the root can create compensatory imbalances (emotional suppression, avoidance).

3. Sustainable healing comes from **metabolic repair**, not just appetite suppression.

📜 Summary

Aspect	Exendin-4–Based (e.g., Byetta)	Human GLP-1–Based (e.g., Semaglutide)
Origin	Gila monster venom protein	Analog of human GLP-1
Risk of Immune Response	High	Low
Gastro Effects	More severe	Milder
Pancreatitis Risk	Elevated	Lower
Duration	Shorter or sustained (Bydureon)	Longer (e.g., once weekly)
Safety Profile	Mixed	Strong clinical data

🔺 RETATRUTIDE OVERVIEW

Retatrutide is a next-generation **triple agonist** targeting:

1. **GLP-1** (Glucagon-Like Peptide-1)

2. **GIP** (Glucose-Dependent Insulinotropic Polypeptide)

3. **Glucagon Receptors**

It is currently in **Phase 2 clinical trials**, showing **unprecedented fat loss results**.

⚙ MECHANISM OF ACTION

Hormone Targeted	Effect
GLP-1	Suppresses appetite, increases insulin, delays gastric emptying
GIP	Improves insulin sensitivity, modulates fat metabolism
Glucagon	Increases energy expenditure, promotes fat burning

🔬 BENEFITS OF RETATRUTIDE

- Up to **24% body weight loss** reported in trials (surpassing semaglutide and tirzepatide).

- Improves **insulin resistance, lipid profiles, and liver fat**.

- Potential future application for **obesity, diabetes, NASH, PCOS**, and metabolic syndrome.

⚠ POTENTIAL RISKS / CONSIDERATIONS

- **More intense side effects** than single or dual agonists: nausea, vomiting, fatigue.

- May cause **lean mass loss** if not paired with protein + resistance training.

- Long-term **glucagon receptor activation** may pose risks to liver health or heart function—still under investigation.

🧬 UPDATED GLP-1 FAMILY COMPARISON TABLE

Peptide	Agonist Targets	Brand Name	Frequency	Relative Potency	Exendin-4?	Notes
Exenatide	GLP-1	Byetta, Bydureon	2x/day (Byetta) or weekly (Bydureon)	Moderate	☑ Yes	Older, immunogenic
Liraglutide	GLP-1	Victoza, Saxenda	Daily	Strong	✕ No	Well-studied
Semaglutide	GLP-1	Ozempic, Wegovy	Weekly	Very strong	✕ No	Gold standard for now
Dulaglutide	GLP-1	Trulicity	Weekly	Strong	✕ No	Once-weekly convenience
Tirzepatide	GLP-1 + GIP	Mounjaro	Weekly	Very strong	✕ No	Superior to semaglutide for weight loss
Retatrutide	GLP-1 + GIP + Glucagon	In trials	Weekly (in studies)	**Most powerful so far**	✕ No	Triple agonist – cutting-edge fat loss

🔑 STRATEGIC USE CASES FOR RETATRUTIDE

Goal	Benefit
Severe obesity or insulin resistance	Rapid and sustained fat loss
Fatty liver / NAFLD	Decreased liver fat and inflammation
Post-PED recovery	Resensitization to insulin, reduced visceral fat
Cognitive clarity	Reduced neuroinflammation and improved metabolic efficiency
Spiritual fasting support	Reduces hunger during detox or intentional restriction cycles

Myostatin Inhibitors and the future of Performance enhancement

Trevogrumab and **Garetosmab** are experimental monoclonal antibodies developed to manipulate key **myostatin-related signaling pathways**. These are at the frontier of **muscle enhancement biotechnology**—offering a glimpse into a future where performance, muscle growth, and even aging could be dramatically altered without traditional anabolic steroids.

1. Trevogrumab (REGN1033)

What It Is:

- A **monoclonal antibody** that **binds to and neutralizes myostatin** (also known as **GDF-8**, a protein that *inhibits muscle growth*).

- Developed by **Regeneron**.

Mechanism:

- Myostatin naturally prevents excessive muscle growth. Trevogrumab **inhibits myostatin**, allowing for increased muscle mass and strength.

Clinical Use Cases Studied:

- **Sarcopenia** (age-related muscle loss)

- **Muscle wasting** in chronic illnesses (e.g., cancer, heart failure)

- **Frailty and disuse atrophy** (e.g., post-surgery, injury)

Status:

- Clinical trials showed **modest increases in muscle mass**, but **less improvement in actual strength or function** than hoped.

- Safety profile still under evaluation.

2. Garetosmab (REGN2477)

What It Is:

- A **monoclonal antibody** that targets **activin A**, a **TGF-beta superfamily protein** also involved in **muscle growth inhibition and inflammation**.

- Also developed by **Regeneron**.

Mechanism:

- Activin A and myostatin **signal through similar pathways (via the ActRIIB receptor)**.

- Blocking activin A may **enhance muscle mass** and **suppress fibrosis or inflammation** in muscular conditions.

Clinical Focus:

- **Fibrodysplasia Ossificans Progressiva (FOP)** — a rare condition where soft tissue turns into bone.

- **Exploration in muscle wasting diseases**, though less publicly studied for athletic enhancement.

FUTURE IMPLICATIONS FOR PERFORMANCE ENHANCEMENT

Potential Benefits

1. **Muscle growth without steroids**

   o Unlike anabolic steroids, these antibodies **do not disrupt hormone systems** directly.

   o Could offer **cleaner, safer hypertrophy** for aging populations or athletes.

2. **Treatment of muscle wasting**

   o Revolutionize care in **cachexia, ALS, sarcopenia**, or **immobility recovery**.

3. **Longer performance careers**

   o Athletes could **maintain muscle mass** well into older age.

   o May reduce injury risk by strengthening supportive musculature.

4. **Space travel & microgravity muscle loss**

   o NASA and similar agencies are investigating these types of therapies for astronauts.

⚠ POSSIBLE RISKS & DOWNSIDES

Risk	Explanation
Excessive hypertrophy	Unchecked muscle growth can strain tendons, fascia, and cardiac function.
Functional imbalance	Some studies showed mass gain without proportional strength or coordination.
Unknown long-term effects	Interfering with growth factors (TGF-beta family) could affect fertility, immunity, or tumor growth.
Ethical abuse in sports	Could become a **black market enhancer** once its effects are better optimized.

🌐 SPIRITUAL & SOCIAL IMPLICATIONS

🌳 Disconnection from Natural Rhythms:

- Relying on external agents to build muscle may reduce **inner discipline**, resilience, or connection to self-earned strength.

Redefining Human Potential:

- Raises questions about **what is "natural" performance**.

- Will **discipline and mastery** be replaced by **biohacks and monoclonal shortcuts**?

Future of Enhancement:

- We're moving toward a paradigm where **gene editing (e.g., CRISPR), antibodies, and peptides** could sculpt the body and mind beyond ancestral limitations.

- The **"transhuman" athlete** may emerge—not just faster and stronger, but longer-lived and fatigue-resistant.

Summary Table

Drug	Target	Purpose	Enhancement Potential
Trevogrumab	Myostatin	Muscle mass gain	Moderate (needs optimization)
Garetosmab	Activin A	Muscle & fibrosis control	Promising (pending further studies)

Chapter 12: The Path of Sacred Strength – What a Healthy Bodybuilding Practice Looks Like

A **Healthy Bodybuilding Lifestyle** that builds **size, strength, and aesthetics** while keeping **hormones, recovery, emotional state, and spiritual alignment** intact.

This isn't just "train and eat clean" — it's a framework where **muscle and mastery** grow together.

⚕ PHYSICAL FOUNDATIONS

1. Smart Training Periodization

- **Cycles of stress and recovery**: alternate hypertrophy, strength, metabolic conditioning, and deload phases.

- Every **8–12 weeks**: reduce volume or intensity to allow joints, tendons, and nervous system to reset.

- Train **with** your circadian rhythm — heavy compound lifts earlier in the day, mobility and restorative work later.

2. Nutrition that Nourishes

- 80% whole-food diet: high-quality protein, varied carbs, essential fats.

- Micronutrient focus: rotate **colorful produce**, use **trace minerals** (magnesium, zinc, copper, selenium).

- Seasonal eating to match **hormonal and immune rhythms**.

- Periodic digestive resets (e.g., 1–2 days of bone broth & easy-to-digest foods).

3. Responsible Enhancement

- If using PEDs or peptides:

  - **On-cycle health support**: antioxidants, liver/kidney support, cardiovascular monitoring.

  - **Bloodwork** every 8–12 weeks.

  - **Post-cycle therapy** to restore natural function.

- Peptide use targeted to recovery, gut health, and longevity (BPC-157, TB-500, MOTS-C, GHK-Cu, Epithalon).

4. Recovery as a Training Pillar

- 7–9 hours of sleep, with deep (delta wave) cycles intact.

- Regular sauna/infrared for circulation & detox.

- Ice baths or cryotherapy for inflammation control after high-load sessions.

- Lymphatic stimulation: rebounder, massage, breathwork.

🧠 MENTAL & EMOTIONAL FOUNDATIONS

1. Purpose Beyond the Mirror

- Set **process-based goals** (strength PRs, mobility gains) alongside aesthetic ones.

- Train for longevity — visualize **lifting at 70+** with quality of life intact.

2. Emotional Awareness

- Recognize when training is a form of **avoidance** vs. **expression**.

- Use movement as **somatic therapy** — consciously release anger, sadness, or tension through intentional sets.

3. Balance Discipline & Flexibility

- Nutrition and training are tools for life, not prison bars.

- Planned indulgences and rest days **prevent rebound binges and burnout**.

⚗ BIOCHEMICAL BALANCE

1. Hormonal Harmony

- Support testosterone naturally with:

  - Adequate fats (omega-3s, saturated fats from clean sources)

  - Micronutrients (zinc, boron, magnesium)

  - Resistance training without chronic overtraining.

- Avoid constant stimulant reliance — use caffeine strategically.

2. Mitochondrial Support

- Use red light therapy, SS-31, MOTS-C, CoQ10, NAD+

- Breath training (nasal breathing, CO_2 tolerance) to optimize oxygen use and Bohr effect.

3. Detox Pathways

- Keep **liver, kidneys, lymphatic system** clear with hydration, greens, cruciferous veggies, sauna, and occasional fasting.

🌱 SPIRITUAL & ENERGETIC ALIGNMENT

1. Training as Ritual

- Treat lifting as a **moving meditation**: focus, breath, intentional movement.

- Pre-lift grounding (breathwork, visualization) to connect with deeper purpose.

2. Integration of Stillness

- Meditation, journaling, or nature walks **balance output with input**.

- Time away from the gym for **creative and relational nourishment**.

3. Respect for the Body as a Temple

- Avoid "punishment workouts" for diet slip-ups.

- Listen to early signs of overtraining — **honor whispers before they become screams**.

🌀 LONG-TERM TRAJECTORY

- Muscular, lean, and functional without sacrificing joint health or hormone stability.

- Psychological flexibility — physique changes don't shatter self-worth.

- Ability to **perform at a high level across decades**, not just for a 5-year competitive window.

- Deep connection to the self, where bodybuilding serves life rather than consuming it.

📜 SUMMARY TABLE

Pillar	Unhealthy Version	Healthy Version
Training	Max effort year-round, no deload	Periodized, planned recovery
Diet	Extreme restriction, poor micronutrients	Nutrient-dense, seasonal, flexible
Enhancement	Max dosages, no breaks	Targeted, monitored, supported
Recovery	Sleep deprivation, no restoration	Sleep, sauna, cold therapy, lymphatic flow
Mindset	Ego-driven, mirror-only goals	Purpose-driven, process-focused
Spirit	Disconnection, avoidance	Integration, reverence for the body

When bodybuilding becomes a **spiritual discipline**:

1. It refines the will, deepens the breath, and grounds the soul in the temple of flesh

2. The barbell becomes a **staff of initiation**

3. The body becomes a **prayer in motion**

✴ **Final Message:** True strength is not in domination, but in devotion. True symmetry is not only of muscle, but of mind, heart, and spirit.

Safe Biomarkers and Spiritual Benchmarks

Depending on your situation and a multitude of factors, what works for one person will vary greatly which is why it is so important to have a professional guide you through this process. If you have spent years competing (like me) you have undoubtedly pushed the limits and amounts of PED's and thrown your body out of balance to achieve the results you desire. No judgement, no shame, I have done it myself which is my purpose for writing this book. The important thing to understand is, there is a good chance your endocrine system requires assistance to stay balanced thus constant monitoring and consistency will any protocol is very important, as this will also dictate your emotional state and spiritual wellness. As we age the body requires more rest and detoxification to heal and recover. Getting bloodwork done every 3-6 months and doing consistent detoxification protocols allows the body to enjoy the benefits of intense training and keeps the mind and body strong and the mind clear.

Balance is key.

The longer one has been using PED's the more likely it is that the receptors are desensitized which is why targeted detoxification and customized bio hacks keep the receptors working efficiently and effectively, and you will feel the difference. Below is a general guideline for things to look for and measure to ensure you are within the ballpark of alignment.

Someone like me, who walked around at 3500 ng/dl of testosterone for five years, I feel sluggish at 750 ng/dl so I prefer to stay around 1200 ng/dl, I also compare those numbers to everything else to make sure nothing is being pushed out of alignment.

Also very important as we get older, and taking testosterone, donate blood every 6 months, as testosterone will increase blood cell count over time. Hematocrit should never get over 55, while 45-48 is optimal. Hematocrit is the thickness of your blood, the thicker it is the more likely blood clots will happen and we don't want those.

Physical Biomarkers to Monitor:

- Testosterone: 750–1200 ng/dL (total), 15–25 pg/mL (free)

Recalibrating Testosterone After Steroid Use

For men who have never interfered with their natural testosterone production, the conventional "optimal" ranges generally serve as a reliable benchmark for health. Yet for those who have spent years cycling anabolic steroids, the journey back to balance is far less straightforward.

After extended periods of supraphysiological testosterone exposure, the body's anabolic receptors become desensitized, and the mind adapts to operating in a state of constant chemical surplus. In this context, returning directly to what is considered a "normal" range may not feel balanced at all. In fact, many men in recovery initially find greater stability at slightly elevated levels while their endocrine system undergoes detoxification and their receptors gradually resensitize. This transition is not merely physiological—it has biochemical and emotional dimensions as well.

Consider a bodybuilder who has lived for years with testosterone levels above 3,000 ng/dL. For him, dropping to 1,700 ng/dL can feel like stepping off a cliff. The nervous system, libido, mood, and sense of identity all require time to recalibrate. The return to equilibrium is best approached as a slow, deliberate process—one that can span months or even years, depending on genetics, lifestyle, cumulative stress, and the psychological adaptations that have been built around an enhanced hormonal state.

In this fragile period, mentorship is invaluable. Having an experienced coach or guide to navigate the complexities of recovery provides not only technical guidance, but also accountability and emotional support. Without such structure, many men either relapse into cycles of abuse or languish in prolonged states of hormonal imbalance.

It's also worth acknowledging that some athletes, after prolonged steroid use, may never fully recover endogenous production to pre-abuse levels. In these cases, testosterone replacement therapy (TRT) may serve as a stabilizing bridge— sometimes temporarily, and in other cases indefinitely. This decision is highly personal, but it is important to remember that *both extremes carry risk*. Low testosterone, just like chronically high testosterone, can have profound consequences for cardiovascular health, cognitive clarity, emotional resilience, and overall vitality.

The ultimate goal, however, is not merely to chase numbers on a blood test. It is to arrive at a sustainable balance—one in which the body is hormonally stable, the mind is emotionally centered, and the spirit can continue its work of growth and integration without being held hostage by chemical swings. This is the path of regenerative bodybuilding: strength pursued in harmony with health, resilience, and self-mastery.

Normal Female Testosterone Ranges

(varies by lab, usually measured in ng/dL)

- **Women (general):** ~15–70 ng/dL

- **Female athletes (naturally high end):** ~50–80 ng/dL

- **On enhancement/TRT (monitored use):** 80–120 ng/dL is sometimes maintained by female bodybuilders for performance.

Optimal for a Female Bodybuilder

- **Target Range:** ~40–80 ng/dL for most women in bodybuilding who are not enhanced.

- This supports:

  o Lean muscle maintenance

  o   Recovery from training

  o   Libido, confidence, and motivation

  o   Bone density and metabolic resilience

- **If enhanced:** some women maintain **80–120 ng/dL** under careful medical supervision — but the higher the level, the higher the risk of masculinization.

⚠ Risks of Supra-Physiological Levels (>120 ng/dL long-term)

- Voice deepening (permanent)

- Hair thinning on scalp, excess body/facial hair

- Menstrual cycle disruption / infertility

- Enlarged clitoris (often irreversible)

- Emotional changes (irritability, volatility)

🧘 Key Considerations for Women in Bodybuilding

1. **Monitor bloodwork regularly** → total testosterone, free testosterone, SHBG, estradiol, DHEA-S.

2. **Support liver and kidney health** if using PEDs or oral AAS (women are more sensitive to hepatotoxicity).

3. **Balance with estrogen and progesterone** → low estradiol can cause joint issues, low mood, and metabolic instability.

4. **Cycle off or use peptides instead** (e.g., IGF-1 LR3, CJC-1295, BPC-157) to support performance without androgenic risks.

5. **Remember longevity** → the goal is strong, lean, and functional long-term, not short-term extremes that compromise femininity or health.

✦ Summary:

For women in bodybuilding, **40–80 ng/dL** is an optimal testosterone range to support performance while staying aligned with health and femininity. Some enhanced athletes may run slightly higher (80–120 ng/dL) for strength and muscle gain, but this must be approached cautiously and monitored closely.

📱 Optimal Estradiol Ranges

Men

- **Typical lab reference range**: ~10–40 pg/mL (37–147 pmol/L)

- **Optimal functional range** (for health, libido, performance):

  - **20–30 pg/mL** (73–110 pmol/L)

- ⚠ Too low (<15 pg/mL):

  - Low libido, joint pain, poor mood, cardiovascular risk.

- ⚠ Too high (>40–50 pg/mL):

  - Water retention, gynecomastia, fat gain (especially around chest/hips), mood swings.

  - Often elevated with anabolic steroid use or obesity/insulin resistance.

Women

Ranges vary by menstrual cycle phase, menopause status, and age.

Phase	Optimal Estradiol (pg/mL)
Follicular (Day 1–13)	~30–120
Ovulatory (Day 14)	~130–370

Luteal (Day 15–28)	~70–250
Postmenopause	<20–30 (unless on HRT)

- ⚠ Too low:

  o Irregular cycles, infertility, low bone density, vaginal dryness, low mood.

- ⚠ Too high:

  o PMS, heavy bleeding, breast tenderness, endometriosis, fibroids, estrogen dominance symptoms.

⏱ Best Time to Test Estradiol

- **Men**: Morning, fasted, alongside testosterone, SHBG, and albumin (to calculate free hormones).

- **Women**:

  o **Day 3 of cycle** (early follicular phase) → baseline estrogen.

  o **Mid-cycle (~Day 14)** if evaluating ovulation.

  o **Day 21** if evaluating luteal phase balance.

⚡ Key Takeaways

- **Men**: Optimal ~20–30 pg/mL. Too high or too low both carry risks.

- **Women**: Highly phase-dependent. Should be interpreted relative to cycle stage or menopausal status.

- Always interpret estradiol with **other hormones** (testosterone, progesterone, LH/FSH, SHBG) for the full picture.

Sex Hormone-Binding Globulin (SHBG) is an important marker for understanding hormone balance, especially in athletes and bodybuilders using PEDs or trying to optimize testosterone function.

🧬 What SHBG Does

- SHBG binds to **sex hormones** (mainly testosterone, dihydrotestosterone, and estradiol).

- Only the **free (unbound) testosterone** and albumin-bound testosterone are biologically active.

- High SHBG → less free T available.

- Low SHBG → more free T, but potentially more hormonal volatility.

🗄 Optimal SHBG Ranges

General Reference Ranges (may vary slightly by lab):
- **Men:** ~15–55 nmol/L

- **Women:** ~30–120 nmol/L

Optimal Range for Male Health & Performance:
- **20–30 nmol/L** is often considered the "sweet spot."

  - Enough SHBG to stabilize hormone fluctuations and protect tissues.

  - Not so high that it traps too much testosterone.

When Too Low (<15 nmol/L):
- Often seen with **insulin resistance, obesity, anabolic steroid use, hypothyroidism**.

- Leads to high free testosterone but more rapid aromatization (→ estrogen conversion).

- Can correlate with **acne, hair loss, and cardiovascular/metabolic risk**.

<u>When Too High (>40–50 nmol/L in men):</u>
- Often linked to **low calorie diets, overtraining, hyperthyroidism, liver disease**.

- Free testosterone becomes very low → fatigue, poor recovery, low libido.

⏰ When to Test SHBG

- **Morning, fasted** (like most hormone labs).

- Avoid heavy training and PED use 24–48 hrs before testing to reduce acute fluctuations.

- Best measured alongside **total testosterone, free testosterone (calculated or direct), estradiol, albumin** for full context.

⚡ Key Insight for Bodybuilders

- **Optimal SHBG** is about **balance**:

  o Too low → lots of free T but instability, faster breakdown, and higher estrogen risk.

  o Too high →" trapped testosterone" with symptoms of low T despite normal totals.

- Staying in that **20–30 nmol/L window** generally provides a good mix of stability and bioavailable testosterone.

Recovering **LH (Luteinizing Hormone)** and **FSH (Follicle Stimulating Hormone)** after years of anabolic steroid use is essentially about rebooting the **hypothalamic–**

---

pituitary–gonadal (HPG) axis. Steroid abuse suppresses this axis because exogenous testosterone (and its derivatives) tell the brain that there's "enough hormone," so the pituitary stops sending LH/FSH to the testes. Over years, this suppression can become semi-permanent without intervention.

Here's a roadmap for how men can optimize recovery:

🧬 Step 1: Assess Baseline Function

- **Labs to Order**:

    o   Total Testosterone, Free Testosterone, SHBG

    o   LH & FSH

    o   Estradiol (E2)

    o   Prolactin

    o   DHEA-S

    o   Thyroid panel (TSH, FT3, FT4) — thyroid dysfunction can worsen HPG suppression

- This helps determine if suppression is **primary (testicular damage)** or **secondary (pituitary/hypothalamic suppression).**

🧬 Step 2: Reboot Strategies

1. SERM Therapy (Selective Estrogen Receptor Modulators)

- **Clomiphene (Clomid)** or **Enclomiphene**

    o   Block estrogen receptors in the hypothalamus → increase GnRH release → pituitary increases LH & FSH.

- **Tamoxifen (Nolvadex)** can also be used in some cases.

Goal: Kickstart the natural signaling of LH/FSH → testicular testosterone and sperm production.

2. hCG (Human Chorionic Gonadotropin) Bridging

- Mimics LH, directly stimulating the testes to produce testosterone.

- Used **before or alongside SERMs** to prevent testicular atrophy if testes are unresponsive.

- Should not be used long-term alone, as it can desensitize LH receptors.

3. Peptide/Gonadotropin Mimetics

- **Kisspeptin-10** or **Kisspeptin-54** → powerful stimulators of GnRH release, potentially resetting the HPG axis.

- **GnRH analog pulsing** can help re-establish pituitary rhythm.

Step 3: Foundational Lifestyle Support

These amplify recovery and prevent relapse into low LH/FSH states:

- **Bodyfat Control**: High visceral fat raises aromatase → higher estrogen → further suppression.

- **Dietary Support**: Zinc, magnesium, boron, vitamin D, omega-3s — all critical for Leydig cell and pituitary function.

- **Sleep & Circadian Rhythm**: Deep sleep is when GnRH pulses occur most strongly.

- **Stress Reduction**: Chronic cortisol elevation suppresses GnRH and pituitary output.

- **Avoid Alcohol & Recreational Drugs**: Direct toxic effects on Leydig and Sertoli cells.

🔄 Step 4: Long-Term Stabilization

- **Slow taper off SERM** once natural T, LH, FSH are in range for several months.

- Monitor every **8–12 weeks** with labs.

- In cases of **permanent suppression or testicular damage**, **long-term TRT** may be necessary.

🧘 Spiritual/Emotional Dimension

- Years of PED use often link self-worth to numbers and physique. The **transition off** can trigger identity crisis, anxiety, or depression.

- Optimizing LH/FSH isn't just about labs — it's about **reclaiming inner balance**, learning to train, eat, and live without external hormonal crutches.

- Breathwork, meditation, and somatic work help reset the nervous system — which is tightly linked to the hypothalamus.

✅ Summary

- **Optimal LH in men**: ~2–10 IU/L

- **Optimal FSH in men**: ~1.5–12 IU/L

- After years of suppression, the path is:

  - **Test baseline → SERM protocol ±hCG → peptides like Kisspeptin (optional) → lifestyle anchoring → taper & stabilize.**

📊 Normal IGF-1 Ranges

(values differ by lab, age, and units; usually ng/mL)

- **Young adults (20s–30s):** ~150–350 ng/mL

- **Middle-aged (40s–50s):** ~100–250 ng/mL
- **Older adults (60+):** ~80–200 ng/mL

HGH abuse can push IGF-1 **well above 400–600 ng/mL**, which increases risk of **insulin resistance, edema, joint issues, heart enlargement, and cancer growth signaling.**

✅ Optimal IGF-1 Targets After PED/HGH Use

- **Goal:** Return IGF-1 to **high-normal for age**, but not supraphysiologic.
- **Optimal Range:**
    - **Men 30–50 years old:** ~150–220 ng/mL
    - **Men 50–60 years old:** ~120–200 ng/mL
- This keeps benefits for **recovery, muscle repair, cognitive health, and metabolism** without overstimulating growth pathways.

⚖️ Why Balance Matters

- **Too Low IGF-1 (<100 ng/mL):**
    - Fatigue, poor recovery, sarcopenia, mood decline, higher frailty risk.
- **Too High IGF-1 (>300–350 ng/mL chronically in adults):**
    - Increases risks of insulin resistance, visceral fat, acromegaly-like features, and long-term cancer promotion.

🛠 Strategies to Optimize IGF-1 Post-PEDs

1. **Rebuild Natural GH Pulsatility**
    - Sleep hygiene (deep sleep = biggest GH pulses).

- o Fasting or time-restricted feeding (improves GH spikes).

- o Exercise (resistance training + HIIT).

2. **Peptides / Secretagogues** (if needed for recovery)

   - o **CJC-1295 (no DAC) + Ipamorelin** → restore natural pulsatile GH release.

   - o **MOTS-C, SS-31** → improve mitochondrial sensitivity to GH/IGF signaling.

   - o **Sermorelin** for more gentle support.

3. **Lifestyle & Nutrition**

   - o Keep **insulin sensitivity high** (low visceral fat, balanced carbs, regular activity).

   - o Adequate protein + micronutrients (zinc, magnesium, vitamin D).

   - o Avoid chronic overfeeding → IGF-1 spikes with excess calories.

4. **Liver Support**

   - o Since IGF-1 is produced in the liver in response to GH, support with:

- NAC, TUDCA, milk thistle, sauna, hydration.

🧘 Spiritual / Emotional Angle

- PED abuse often represents a phase of **pushing growth unnaturally**.

- Restoring IGF-1 to a **balanced range** mirrors the spiritual principle of **sufficiency** — honoring the body's natural rhythm rather than forcing more.

- A healthy IGF-1 means the body is in a state of **repair, renewal, and harmony**, not overgrowth or depletion.

Summary:

After years of HGH and PED abuse, aim for **IGF-1 levels in the 150–220 ng/mL range (for men under 50)** or **120–200 ng/mL (for older men)**. This supports recovery and vitality without reigniting the risks associated with supraphysiologic IGF-1.

Core Bloodwork (Liver Function Tests – LFTs)

1. **ALT (Alanine Aminotransferase)**

   o Key enzyme indicating hepatocellular injury.

   o Elevated = liver cell damage.

2. **AST (Aspartate Aminotransferase)**

   o Also reflects liver cell damage, but less specific than ALT.

   o AST:ALT ratio can help identify alcoholic liver disease vs. other causes.

3. **ALP (Alkaline Phosphatase)**

   o Elevated in **bile duct obstruction** or gallbladder issues.

4. **GGT (Gamma-Glutamyl Transferase)**

   o Sensitive for **biliary tract health** and alcohol-related liver stress.

   o Helps confirm whether ALP elevation is liver-related vs. bone-related.

5. **Bilirubin (Total & Direct)**

   o Indicates bile metabolism and excretion efficiency.

   o Elevated = obstruction, hemolysis, or liver dysfunction.

6. **Albumin**

   o Protein made by the liver; low levels may indicate chronic liver disease.

7. **Prothrombin Time (PT/INR)**

   o   Measures clotting factor production (made in the liver).

   o   Prolonged PT = advanced liver dysfunction.

Extended / Functional Markers

8. **LDH (Lactate Dehydrogenase)**

   o   Non-specific, but sometimes elevated in liver injury.

9. **Ferritin & Iron Studies**

   o   Detects hemochromatosis (iron overload → liver damage).

10. **Ceruloplasmin & Copper**

- For Wilson's disease (rare, copper accumulation).

11. **Lipid Panel**

- Dyslipidemia often coexists with fatty liver.

12. **Fasting Insulin & HbA1c**

- Insulin resistance is strongly tied to NAFLD (fatty liver disease).

Imaging

- **Ultrasound** → baseline screening for fatty liver, gallstones, bile duct dilation.

- **FibroScan (elastography)** → measures liver stiffness to detect fibrosis.

- **MRI/CT** → if deeper imaging is needed.

When to Test

- **Baseline** if you have a history of PEDs, alcohol, high-protein diets, or long-term meds.

- **Every 3–6 months** if enhanced or using hepatotoxic compounds (oral steroids, SARMs, high-dose supplements, alcohol).

- **Annually** for general health if no major risks.

🧘 Key Takeaway

The most **critical blood markers** for liver health are:

ALT, AST, ALP, GGT, Bilirubin, Albumin, and PT/INR.

From there, add iron studies, fasting insulin, and imaging for a more complete picture.

🔑 Key Gallbladder-Related Markers

1. **Alkaline Phosphatase (ALP)**

   o Elevated in **bile duct obstruction** or sluggish bile flow (cholestasis).

   o A primary marker for gallbladder stress when combined with other tests.

2. **Gamma-Glutamyl Transferase (GGT)**

   o Very sensitive to **biliary tract dysfunction**.

   o Helps confirm if an ALP rise is from gallbladder/bile ducts (and not bone turnover).

3. **Bilirubin (Total & Direct)**

   o Elevated levels suggest bile is not flowing properly (gallstones, duct obstruction).

   o **Direct bilirubin** rises when bile ducts are blocked.

4. **ALT & AST (Liver Enzymes)**

   ○ Elevated if there's secondary liver irritation from gallbladder or bile duct issues.

   ○ Not gallbladder-specific, but important in the overall picture.

Functional or Additional Markers

- **Serum Lipase/Amylase** → May rise if gallbladder dysfunction irritates the pancreas.

- **Cholesterol Profile** → Bile is made from cholesterol; imbalances can indicate poor bile metabolism.

- **FibroTest / FibroSure (advanced panels)** → Evaluate fibrosis risk if chronic bile obstruction is suspected.

Summary

For gallbladder health in a **bloodwork panel**, the most useful markers are:

- **ALP + GGT + Bilirubin** → core trio for gallbladder/bile duct health.

- Supporting: **ALT, AST, Lipase** → to check secondary effects on liver/pancreas.

- Lipid panel for functional insight.

If you want a **single most useful marker**, **GGT** is often considered the most **sensitive for gallbladder/biliary stress**, especially when interpreted alongside ALP and bilirubin.

Key Kidney Markers for Bodybuilders

Basic Kidney Panel

1. **Serum Creatinine**

   o Byproduct of muscle metabolism.

   o Elevated in bodybuilders even without kidney damage (due to high muscle mass + creatine use).

   o Needs context with other markers.

2. **Blood Urea Nitrogen (BUN)**

   o Reflects protein metabolism and kidney excretion.

   o Can rise with high protein diets — not always pathology by itself.

3. **eGFR (Estimated Glomerular Filtration Rate)**

   o Calculated from creatinine.

   o Can underestimate kidney function in muscular individuals (false low).

Advanced / More Accurate Markers

4. **Cystatin C**

   o Better kidney marker in athletes because it isn't affected by muscle mass.

   o Provides a more accurate eGFR when combined with creatinine.

5. **Urine Albumin-to-Creatinine Ratio (ACR)**

   o Detects **early kidney stress/damage** before serum creatinine rises.

   o Key for catching kidney strain from PEDs or long-term high protein intake.

6. **Urinalysis (Dipstick or Microscopy)**

   o   Looks for protein, blood, or crystals in urine.

   o   Can identify rhabdomyolysis risk or stone formation.

7. **Electrolytes (Sodium, Potassium, Chloride, Bicarbonate)**

   o   Important when using **diuretics, cutting agents, or dehydration tactics**.

8. **Phosphorus & Calcium**

   o   Imbalances can reflect kidney stress or altered bone-mineral handling.

⏱ Optimal Timing for Bloodwork

- **Best Time of Day**:

   o   Morning, fasted, hydrated with just water.

   o   Avoid training, supplements, or protein meals before testing (they can skew results).

- **Avoid Pre-Test Confounders** (24–48 hrs before):

   o   Intense workouts (can elevate creatinine, CK, and protein in urine).

   o   Very high protein meals.

   o   Creatine supplements (pause 2–3 days if possible).

   o   Dehydration (concentrates BUN/creatinine, giving false positives).

- **Frequency**:

   o   At least **2–3x per year** for bodybuilders using PEDs, diuretics, or high protein intake.

- Every **8–12 weeks** if on cycle, especially with orals, NSAIDs, or other kidney-stressing agents.

⚡ Summary

- **Must-haves**: Creatinine, BUN, eGFR, urinalysis.

- **Best practice for athletes**: Add **Cystatin C + ACR** for accuracy.

- **Optimal timing**: Morning, fasted, hydrated, after 1–2 days of lighter training & moderate protein intake.

- **Frequency**: 2–3x/year minimum; every cycle if enhanced.

Core Thyroid Panel

1. **TSH (Thyroid-Stimulating Hormone)**

   - Standard screening test.

   - High TSH = underactive thyroid, low TSH = overactive or suppressed.

   - But **TSH alone is not enough** — PEDs and stress can distort it.

2. **Free T4 (Thyroxine)**

   - The main thyroid hormone released from the gland.

   - Measures *circulating available T4*, not just bound hormone.

3. **Free T3 (Triiodothyronine)**

   - The active thyroid hormone inside cells.

   - PED use, stress, and calorie restriction often reduce T4→T3 conversion.

🔬 Advanced Thyroid Markers

4. **Reverse T3 (rT3)**

   o Inactive form of T3 produced under stress, inflammation, or high cortisol.

   o High rT3 = blocked thyroid activity at the cellular level ("thyroid resistance").

5. **Total T3 and Total T4**

   o Gives context to free hormone levels, especially if SHBG or albumin is altered by PEDs.

6. **Thyroid Antibodies** (to rule out autoimmune issues triggered by stress or PED use):

   o **Anti-TPO (Thyroid Peroxidase Antibodies)**

   o **Anti-Tg (Thyroglobulin Antibodies)**

   o Elevated = Hashimoto's or autoimmune thyroiditis risk.

⚡ Supporting Markers (Metabolic Context)

- **Cortisol (AM serum or DUTCH test)** → high cortisol blocks T4→T3 conversion.

- **Ferritin & Iron Panel** → iron deficiency disrupts thyroid hormone production.

- **Vitamin D, Zinc, Selenium, Magnesium** → key cofactors for thyroid function.

- **Lipid Panel** → hypothyroidism often raises cholesterol and triglycerides.

⏱ When to Test

- **Morning, fasted** for the most accurate thyroid readings.

- **Avoid stimulants** (caffeine, clenbuterol, fat burners) the morning of bloodwork.

- Ideally after a **week off PEDs or thermogenics** if possible, since these can artificially skew results.

Key Takeaway

For optimal thyroid recovery after PED use, the best panel includes:

- **TSH, Free T4, Free T3, Reverse T3, Anti-TPO, Anti-Tg.**

- Add **cortisol, ferritin, and micronutrient tests** for the full metabolic picture.

Spiritual Biomarkers (less measurable but equally important):

- Emotional resilience

- Presence in the gym, not dissociation

- Ability to rest without guilt

- Relationship to food and body image

- Willingness to listen to pain as guidance

Emotional Resilience

How to Evaluate:

- Notice how you respond when things don't go to plan: missed lifts, injuries, bad sleep, or setbacks outside the gym.

- Do you collapse into frustration and self-criticism, or can you adapt, breathe, and redirect?

Tools:

- Keep a **resilience journal**: note situations that trigger you and how you responded.

- Reflect weekly on whether you recovered faster emotionally than before.

🏋️ Presence in the Gym, Not Dissociation

How to Evaluate:

- Track how often you enter a "flow state" where you feel connected to breath, form, and muscle engagement.

- Ask yourself: *Do I train with awareness, or do I mentally check out while chasing numbers?*

Tools:

- Practice **mind–muscle connection scans** mid-set — sensing contraction and release.

- Use a **1–10 awareness scale** after workouts: how present were you?

😌 Ability to Rest Without Guilt

How to Evaluate:

- Notice if you can take a rest day, deload week, or nap without anxiety about "losing progress."

- Do you equate rest with laziness, or with integration and growth?

Tools:

- Journal before rest: write down what guilt arises.

- Reframe rest as part of discipline, not absence of it.

- Reflect: *Do I feel recharged after rest, or restless and ashamed?*

🍽 Relationship to Food and Body Image

How to Evaluate:

- Pay attention to how you view meals: are they fuel and nourishment, or do you feel stress, shame, or obsession?

- Notice body-checking behaviors: how often do you critique yourself in the mirror?

Tools:

- Use mindful eating practices: chew slowly, notice taste, gratitude for the food.

- Rate post-meal feelings: satisfaction, guilt, or anxiety?

- Journal body image reflections weekly, noting shifts toward acceptance or criticism.

⚠ Willingness to Listen to Pain as Guidance

How to Evaluate:

- Track how you respond to pain signals: do you push through, mask with stimulants, or pause and investigate?

- Distinguish "good" pain (muscle fatigue, growth) from "warning" pain (joint, nerve, sharp or chronic).

Tools:

- After each session, do a **body scan meditation**: listen to subtle signals of strain or imbalance.

- Keep a "pain journal" noting when pain arose, what action you took, and what outcome followed.

✦ Pulling it All Together

Create a **Spiritual Biomarker Check-in** once a week:

1. How resilient was I this week?

2. Was I present in my lifts?

3. Did I allow myself rest without guilt?

4. How did I relate to food and my body?

5. Did I listen to pain, or override it?

This check-in becomes your **inner bloodwork** — a way to measure growth in **spirit and mind** alongside growth in muscle.

Peptide Optimization Dosage Calculator

Peptide	Primary Benefit	Recommended Dosage	Timing Protocol
Thymosin Alpha 1	Immune modulation	1.6–2.0 mg	2–3x/week subQ
Thymosin Beta 4	Tissue repair, anti-inflammatory	2–5 mg	2–3x/week subQ
BPC-157	Gut, tendon, nerve healing	200–500 mcg	1–2x/day subQ or oral (for gut)
Epithalon	Telomere support, longevity	5–10 mg	1x/day for 10–20 days; 2–3x/year
SS-31	Mitochondrial protection	5–10 mg	1x/day subQ or IV
GHK-Cu	Skin, hair, tissue healing	2–5 mg	Topical or subQ daily
DSIP	Deep sleep support	100–300 mcg	Before bed, subQ or intranasal

Semax	Cognition, neuroprotection	300–600 mcg	2–3x/day intranasal
Selank	Anti-anxiety, mood	250–500 mcg	2–3x/day intranasal
Dihexa	Neurogenesis, memory	8–12 mg	Oral, 1x/day; cycling recommended
IGF-1 LR3	Muscle growth, recovery	20–50 mcg	Pre/post workout, subQ or IM
Sermorelin	GH release	200–500 mcg	Before bed, subQ (5x/week)
Ibutamoren (MK-677)	GH/IGF-1 boost	10–25 mg	Oral 1x/day, PM preferred
CJC-1295 (w/ DAC)	GH release (long acting)	1–2 mg	2x/week subQ
Tesamorelin	Visceral fat reduction	2 mg	1x/day subQ
MOTS-C	Metabolic optimization	5–15 mg	1x/day subQ, 2–4 weeks on
-ARA 290.00	Nerve healing, anti-inflammatory	4 mg	1x/day subQ
LL-37	Antimicrobial, immune	100–500 mcg	1x/day subQ, pulse cycle
Slu-pp-332	Fat loss, metabolism	TBD (research only)	Experimental use only